CU00841224

Knee Arthritis: Take Back Control

From Exercises to Knee Replacements & Everything In Between

Chloe Wilson

Wilson Health Ltd
5 Minton Place
Victoria Road,
Bicester, Oxon
OX26 6QB

Contents

Disclaimer

Introduction

Arthritis is the leading cause of disability in the US and affects millions of people worldwide. In 2009, osteoarthritis was the 4th most frequent reason for hospital stays in the US[1].

For many, the diagnosis of arthritis is a scary prospect and many people don't get the help they need. Little information is shared and common myths abound. Images are conjured in our minds of bones crumbling and life in a wheelchair. Forget playing sport or doing the activities that you love, life as you know it is over. Many people aren't ever given the option to see a specialist health professional. For some who are, it may simply not be affordable and for others, life is just too busy. To many, the simplest solution is to avoid anything that hurts or might cause further damage, just cross your fingers and hope it doesn't get any worse.

But this doesn't have to be the case. With the information you will find here in this book, you can take back control. You can arm yourself with knowledge and understanding of what is going on, and equip yourself to get your knee to the best state possible. Don't get me wrong, there is no magic cure for arthritis. You can't wave a magic wand and it all go away. But, there is a lot that you can do to improve the function of your knee and reduce, maybe even abolish, the pain that you get.

In the first part of this book, we will look in-depth at what happens in the knee with arthritis and how to overcome the pain and debilitation it so often causes. There are many ways to overcome the problems associated with knee arthritis and for most people, these will be enough. However, some will require surgical intervention, and as such, the second half of this book looks at the surgical options concentrating on the most common - knee replacements. In both parts, you will find out everything you need to know and how you can get the best from your knee. You will be amazed by how much difference you can make to your own recovery, by understanding what is going on, making a few simple changes and using my top tips.

I worked as a physiotherapist for over ten years and have seen countless patients with arthritis and recovering from knee replacements. Here I will share with you my knowledge and experience, in an easy to follow and understand format to demystify the medical jargon so often used.

Now, before you go any further it is important that you remember this. This book is aimed at the general public but should in no way delay or substitute medical advice. Before you start using any of the principles outlined here, please see your doctor to check what is appropriate for you. Everyone's situation is different. Once you've got the all clear, off you go! So let's begin.

Chapter 1. What Is Knee Arthritis?

So what is arthritis? "Arthritis" is a blanket term which simply means "inflammation of the joint". There are actually over a hundred different types of arthritis and associated conditions, but the two most common categories that affect the knee joint are caused by either "wear and tear", e.g. Osteoarthritis, or "inflammation" e.g. Rheumatoid Arthritis. Let's have a quick look at each of these.

Osteoarthritis (OA)

What is It? Wear and tear of the bones and cartilage in the knee

Causes: Previous knee injury or surgery, being overweight, genetics, gender, aging

Symptoms: Often fluctuate and may include stiffness (especially in the morning), pain, swelling, weakness and instability

This is commonly known as "wear and tear" arthritis and is by far the most common cause of arthritis pain in knees. Approximately 13% of women and 10% of men aged 60 years and older have symptomatic knee OA[2] (meaning that it is causing them symptoms such as pain and swelling), and there are many more who have OA but are unaware of it (asymptomatic). Studies have shown there is little correlation between the symptoms felt with OA and the amount of damage seen on x-ray – more on this in chapter 4.

Rheumatoid Arthritis

What Is It? A long term condition causing joint inflammation and destruction that can affect any part of the body

Causes: Autoimmune disease – the body starts attacking itself, the trigger of which is unknown

Symptoms: Throbbing/aching pain, swelling, redness and stiffness in joints, usually affecting both sides of the body (e.g. both hands). Symptoms may come and go with periods of "flare-ups"

Rheumatoid arthritis is a chronic, systemic inflammatory disorder. Simply put, it means this: chronic = long term, systemic = throughout the body, inflammatory = swelling. With rheumatoid arthritis, your body mistakenly sends antibodies (which should normally attack bacteria and viruses) to attack the tissues lining the surfaces of joints in the body such as the knee. Chemicals are released causing inflammation and excessive fluid production in the joints which in turn damages nearby bones and soft tissues including cartilage. Joints become swollen, painful and warm, movement is limited by resultant stiffness and over time, the joints may become deformed.

Rheumatoid arthritis is less common than osteoarthritis and its incidence is actually declining. It affects around 1% of the world's population and is three times more prevalent in women than men. Onset usually occurs between the ages of 40-50. It will usually affect a number of joints, especially the hands, feet and neck. Symptoms can come and go, known as "flare ups". One of the most distinguishing features is joint stiffness following periods of inactivity (such as sleeping) which eases with movement.

In this book, we are going to concentrate on osteoarthritis as this is by far the most common type of arthritis affecting the knee. From here on in, when you see the word "arthritis", it is referring to Osteoarthritis.

Chapter 2. What Is Going On?

Let's start by taking a quick look at the anatomy of the knee joint so we can understand what goes wrong in arthritis. The knee is the largest and one of the most complex joints in the human body. The knee joint is typically thought of as where the thigh bone (femur) and shin bone (tibia) meet, medically referred to as the tibiofemoral joint. This is a hinge joint which means it can bend, straighten and twist slightly.

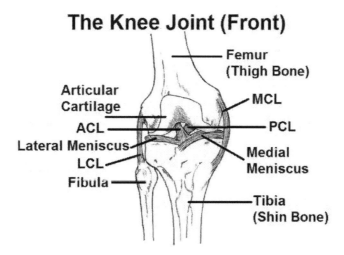

The surface of the bones are lined with articular cartilage, and the joint is surrounded by a small sac, known as the joint capsule. This contains synovial fluid which lubricates the joint. There is an extra layer of thick, rubbery cartilage on the top surface of the tibia, known as the meniscus. This works as a shock absorber to reduce the forces going through the knee. It is divided into two parts, the medial meniscus (on the inner side)

and the lateral meniscus (on the outer side). There are four ligaments which help stabilise the knee. Inside the joint are the anterior and posterior cruciate ligaments (ACL and PCL) and on either side of the joint are the medial and lateral collateral ligaments (MCL and LCL).

In a normal, healthy knee joint, there is a reasonable sized gap between the two knee bones due to the thick layer of cartilage and lubricating (synovial) fluid. The surface of the bones are nice and smooth so as the knee bends/straightens, the joint moves easily and painlessly due to this cushioning effect.

With osteoarthritis of the knee, a few things happen. Changes in the collagen matrix in the cartilage cause it to thin and break down and as a result the bone underneath begins to thicken and lays down new bone to try and protect itself. These spurs stick up so the joint surfaces are no longer smooth but are a bit bumpy. They are known as osteophytes or knee bone spurs. Synovial fluid loses its viscosity and there may also be inflammation of the joint capsule, and thickening of the ligaments.

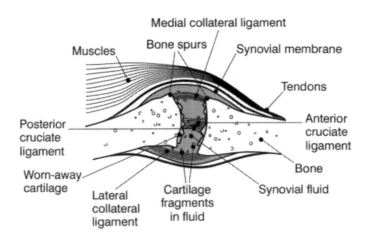

As a result of these changes, there is less space between the bones. This means that as you use the knee, you can get friction in the joint with bone rubbing on bone. The bone spurs can also limit the amount of movement in the knee leading to stiffness.

Arthritis may occur throughout the knee or just on one side of the joint, most commonly on the inner side.

10 Second Summary

Osteoarthritis is when degeneration of the cartilage and bones lead to bony lumps forming. These lumps limit movement and cause pain.

Chapter 3: Causes of OA Knee

There is usually no one specific cause of OA but there are a number of factors which have been found to be linked with the condition. Let's have a look at the seven most common factors:

1) Age

Arthritis is related to, but not entirely caused by, aging, most commonly affecting people over the age of 65. As we age, our bones become more brittle, our muscles often weaken, and the body becomes less efficient at healing itself. As a result, the cartilage and bone are more prone to damage, resulting in arthritis in the knee. About 10% of people aged over 55 years have painful, disabling knee OA, of whom a quarter are severely disabled[3].

2) Weight

Studies have shown that osteoarthritis is three times more likely in people who are overweight (BMI over 27). There are a number of theories behind this. One is that the more we weigh, the more weight goes through our bones, and therefore the more likely that the cartilage will get worn away. Another is that obesity can also lead to changes in metabolic factors and secretion of active agents such as adipocytokines which lead to joint degradation and inflammation[4].

However, it is not as simple as saying that if you are overweight you will get arthritis in the knee but there is a direct correlation.

3) Gender

Women are almost twice as likely to develop arthritis in the knee as men[5]. There are two likely reasons for this. Firstly, women's hormone levels affect the cartilage and bone, especially after the menopause. Secondly, wider hips make subtle changes to the knee position making it more prone to wear and tear.

4) Previous Injury

Previous damage to the knee can also increase your risk of developing arthritis. Let me give you a few examples. Meniscus tears often don't heal properly due to a poor blood supply and this increases the risk of wear and tear in the joint. Ligament tears can affect the stability of the knee which can increase the forces through the joint, increasing the likelihood of arthritis. Fractures also increase the risk as when the broken bone heals it will never be exactly the same as it was before.

5) Previous Surgery

Studies have shown that if you have had part of your cartilage removed in the past (known as a meniscectomy), you are more likely to develop arthritis in the knee[6] This is most likely a result of the fact that the cartilage never regrows, which puts more pressure and friction through the bones. It is thought that the more cartilage is removed, the higher the incidence of knee arthritis in the longer term.

6) Biomechanics

Studies have shown a link between malalignment at the knee and arthritis[7]. This is because changes in position can affect how the forces go through the knee. In a normal knee, 60-70% of the load goes through the medial (inner) side of the knee. Any shift in either direction affects the distribution of the load. These changes may be genetic, due to factors such as muscle imbalance (weakness/tightness) or altered foot position e.g. flat feet.

7) Genetics

While we don't fully understand the link between genes and arthritis, studies looking at family cohorts and twins have produced strong evidence that a link exists. One example of this is that our genes may affect the make-up of our cartilage[8] - some people are born with amazing quality cartilage, others like me aren't! Another is a specific pattern of gene variations in the IL1RN gene, which is involved in controlling inflammation, making it more likely that arthritis will progress to being more severe[9].

Chapter 4: Diagnosis & Symptoms

Your doctor can normally diagnose arthritis by talking to you about your symptoms and examining the knee. They may also arrange for x-rays to confirm or deny the diagnosis. X-rays may show decreased joint space (the distance between the bones), increased bone formation around the joint (known as subchondral sclerosis), subchondral cysts and osteophytes.

Symptoms can be split into two different groups:

1) Subjective Findings: These are the symptoms felt by the affected individual. One example of this is the pain felt, including the location, severity (often on a scale of 0-10) and nature (e.g. sharp or dull)

2) Objective Findings: These are verifiable indications that can be seen, heard, felt and measured. With arthritis, this includes things like the level of cartilage & bone degeneration found on x-ray and range of movement at the knee

Surprisingly, there is often very little correlation between the two. For example, some people demonstrate advanced arthritis on x-ray but have minimal symptoms, whereas other people suffering from a great deal of pain may only show mild changes on x-ray.

Medically speaking, OA can be categorised into three stages.

Stage 1: Mild Arthritis

The technical term for this stage is "Early Degenerative Changes".

Objective findings: X-rays will usually show minimal changes to the bone and cartilage. Range of movement is usually not affected, or only very mildly.

Subjective Findings: Symptoms usually start with a generalised ache around the knee. Stiffness can occur especially after prolonged periods in one position e.g. after sitting, when getting up in the morning or after lots of exercise. People often get pain when going down stairs or getting up from a chair. In this stage, there may be no significant symptoms at all and arthritis often goes undiagnosed as a result.

Stage 2: Moderate Arthritis

The technical term for this stage is "Moderately Advanced Arthritis".

Objective Findings: X-rays will often show narrowing of the joint space (the gap between the bones) and loss of the smooth surface of the bones with some osteophyte formation - bony knee spurs. The knee may start to swell and/or stiffen. It may not be able to bend and straighten fully and sometimes the joint starts to make funny noises e.g. creaking or cracking noises. Muscle weakness may develop due to decreased activity levels.

Subjective Findings: Pain and stiffness, especially first thing in the morning or after sitting for prolonged periods. These usually ease with movement. Activities of daily living may be affected and there may be a feeling of not quite trusting the knee.

Stage 3: Severe Arthritis

The technical term for this stage is "Advanced Arthritis".

Objective Findings: X-rays may show complete loss of joint space with a number of osteophytes. The range of movement at the knee will likely be decreased (loss of end range flexion and extension) and there may be audible and palpable crepitus (a grating sound or sensation produced by friction between the bones/cartilage). The knee can also become deformed.

Subjective Findings: Arthritis knee pain can end up so severe that normal daily activities such as walking and going down stairs become extremely painful and difficult. Sleep may also be affected due to the pain.

When planning treatment, it is much more important to concentrate on your symptoms, rather than what your x-ray shows.

Symptoms Of Arthritis

Let's look in a bit more detail at the common symptoms experienced with osteoarthritis. Knee arthritis symptoms vary greatly from person to person and even day to day. Some days there may be no pain at all, other days you may be in agony.

1) Pain

Pain is the most common complaint and is typically felt when trying to fully bend or straighten the knee e.g. squatting and with activities where lots of weight goes through the knee e.g. going up and down stairs or running. The knee is often sore when you touch it. Pain levels tend to fluctuate. People often describe arthritis pain as being like a "nagging toothache".

2) Stiffness

Another one of the most common knee arthritis symptoms is stiffness which limits how much you can bend and straighten your knee. Stiffness first thing in the morning or after prolonged inactivity e.g. sitting for long periods is a classic feature of arthritis. The stiffness usually eases after a few minutes of moving around. Doing gentle exercises when you first wake up or when you are sitting can really help reduce this stiffness (more on this in Chapter 8).

3) Swelling

Knee swelling is another common feature of arthritis. Irritation at the joint from wear and tear can lead to increased production of synovial fluid and therefore swelling. The swelling tends to fluctuate and can cause pain and restricted movement. Ice and Tubigrip compression bandage can really help to reduce the swelling associated with arthritis.

4) Fluctuating Symptoms

People often find their symptoms vary greatly. Some days they feel fine, other days they are in complete agony. Symptoms are often worse during:

a) Bad weather: the thinking behind this is that the change in air pressure affects the pressure in our joints

b) When we are stressed/anxious/tired: During these times chemicals are released in our body that make us feel pain more

c) When we are unwell: inflammatory chemicals are often released into our system when we are ill, increasing arthritis knee pain

5) Weakness & Instability

Sometimes arthritis can cause weakness and instability around the knee, and the knee may give way at times. This tends to be the result of you using the knee less due to pain and stiffness – the more it hurts, the less we do causing muscles to lose strength and flexibility.

The Arthritis Vicious Cycle

A vicious cycle often develops with OA. Arthritis causes pain so you stop moving the knee as much. Then as a result the knee gets stiffer, and you lose more movement. When you then try and move the knee, it hurts more, so you stop using it and the cycle continues in a downward spiral. The same goes for the strength of the knee.

If activities start feeling painful, we tend to avoid them, but then the muscles get weaker. As a result they can't support the joint and more weight ends up going through the bones and things get more painful. Yet another vicious cycle. This is why exercises are one of the best arthritis treatment options. Muscles only stay strong by being used.

10 Second Summary

There are three stages of knee arthritis. While they generally show progressive symptoms of pain and stiffness, there may be little correlation between the amount of actual damage to the bone and cartilage and the symptoms felt.

Chapter 5: Arthritis Treatment Options

Knee arthritis treatment aims to reduce pain, increase function and slow/halt the progression of the disease.

It is important to remember that there is no cure for arthritis, the changes in the bone and cartilage cannot be undone. But the effect of those changes can be minimised. The ultimate goal is to enable you to manage your symptoms so you can get on with your life. By reducing pain and swelling, and improving the strength and mobility of your knee, you can improve your day to day life.

There is no magic formula for treating arthritis, different things will work for different people at different times. It's about finding the right combination for you.

Conventional Treatment For Knee Arthritis

SAFETY ADVICE: Always discuss any new knee arthritis treatment with your doctor first to make sure it is appropriate for you.

1) Exercise

Once upon a time people were told that exercise made arthritis worse. Nothing could be further from the truth. Studies have consistently shown that one of the best treatments for mild and moderate OA knee is exercise[10]. Ideally you want a combination of aerobic exercises like swimming and cycling combined with strengthening and mobility exercises.

a) Strengthening Exercises: Stronger muscles means more support for the knee and therefore less force through the bones resulting in less pain

b) Mobility Exercises: when the knee starts getting stiff and the muscles get tight, it can change the way forces go through the knee and can put extra pressure on the cartilage and bones. Walking on a leg that doesn't fully straighten, even just by a few degrees, is much harder work

If you are a keen runner and suffer from arthritis, it's best to avoid hard running surfaces like pavements. Instead opt for a treadmill, cross trainer, or grass.

2) Medication

This may be over-the-counter treatment or prescription medications. I know a lot of people don't like taking pills but they can be really useful. It is generally much better to take pain relief in the short term so that you can keep active and do exercises than it is to battle through pain while your knee gets weaker and more painful.

Your doctor may recommend simple painkillers such as paracetamol or anti-inflammatories such as Non-Steroidal Anti-Inflammatory Drugs (NSAID). Some are available over the counter e.g. ibuprofen/Advil and stronger ones are available on prescription. NSAIDs work by reducing swelling and pain.

Please remember, always consult your doctor before taking any medication as there are some side effects and contraindications associated with certain drugs.

3) Heat/Ice

Heat: warmth to an arthritic joint can be very soothing and is a lovely, natural treatment. The heat sensation can help to block out the pain and also helps increase blood flow to the area. This brings in oxygen, chemicals and nutrients that the joint needs to heal whilst at the same time taking away the waste products that can be irritating the joint and contributing to the pain. Heat can also help to reduce muscle spasms.

The simplest ways to apply heat are to either use a hot water bottle (ensuring it has a fluffy cover or a towel wrapped around it), or a microwaveable wheat bag and use for up to 15-20 minutes at a time. Always use with care to ensure you don't overheat the area or burn yourself.

Ice: ice can also help reduce pain and swelling, by reducing the blood flow to the area, known as vasoconstriction. Ice may be more useful during flare-up periods with arthritis. There are a number of different ways to apply ice including ice bags, instant ice packs or cryocuffs. Ice should never be placed directly on the skin, as there is a risk of developing an ice burn. It should be used for 10-15 minutes at a time leaving a couple of hours in between applications. If ice is left on too long, it can actually make things worse as if the area gets too cold, the blood vessels actually widen, known as cold induced vasodilation, rather than constricting which can increase swelling!

SAFETY ADVICE: Never use heat or ice if you have any problems with the sensation in your knee, circulation problems or diabetes or over an open wound or stitches.

4) Keep Moving

Our joints need movement. As we mentioned in chapter 2, the knee joint is surrounded by a bag like structure (known as the joint capsule) which contains fluid which works to lubricate the joint – think of it like the oil in your car which keeps everything moving smoothly. The fluid is pumped into the joint with movement of the knee.

However, if the knee remains in one position for too long, the fluid starts to "dry out" and the knee loses some of its lubrication. This is why when you go to get up in the morning or after sitting down for a while the knee feels stiff and sore, but then loosens up after a few minutes. Therefore, try and avoid staying still for long periods. Every twenty minutes or so, do some simple exercises like bending and straightening your leg (more on this in chapter 8). And before you get up in the morning, do some exercises to help loosen the knee and get the fluid pumping back in to the joint – it will make those first few steps a little easier.

5) Activity Modification & Pacing

Making some simple changes to how you carry out your activities can make a big difference with arthritis. Rather than spending a long time on certain activities or trying to do everything in one day, pace your activities through the day – don't try and do all the strenuous jobs at once. Alternate between physical activities and gentler ones. If you can, change your position for activities, maybe sitting for activities when you would classically stand, or getting up every twenty minutes or so if you are doing a seated activity like working on the computer. Organise your day so you don't have to go up and downstairs too many times, and when you do, use the handrail or go one step at a time.

Keep using your knee, but rest when it becomes painful. Split activities across the week. As I have said, symptoms often vary day to day with arthritis and it can be tempting to overdo things on your good days. This often leads to a boom and bust cycle where when you feel good you do loads, but then you pay for it the next day. Little and often works much better. If you pace yourself properly so you can keep going, you will find you get more done over the course of a week, rather than overdoing it one day and being knocked out the next.

6) Injections

There are two types of injections that can be helpful for knee arthritis.

Corticosteroid injections are a mixture of local anaesthetic and steroid that is injected into the joint to help decrease pain and swelling. The benefits are usually felt almost immediately and may last for a few months.

Joint lubricant injections such as Synvisc, involve injecting a natural gel-like substance found in normal joints into the knee to help lubricate it, as well as decreasing inflammation. It can take a few weeks to notice the effects.

These injections are often carried out by your own doctor. Whilst they won't cure your arthritis, they may relieve pain for up to 6 months. However, injections should never be used in isolation as a treatment for arthritis, they should be combined with other treatments.

7) Weight Loss & Diet

Research has shown that reducing body weight by 5-10% can considerably reduce arthritis knee pain. Each pound of weight lost results in a 4-fold reduction in the load exerted on the knee per step with daily activities[11]. It can also improve your ability to carry out exercise. However, weight loss is only recommended as part of knee arthritis treatment if you are overweight so always consult your doctor before embarking on a weight loss programme.

There are also certain foods that it is worth avoiding with arthritis as well as some that can help. By making good arthritis food choices, you can help reduce inflammation and pain. We will look at this in Chapter 7.

8) Walking Aids

Sometimes people with OA knee find it helpful to use a stick or crutches. Crutches can be used to reduce how much weight is going through the knee when we walk. A stick doesn't really take any weight off the joint but it does help you to balance.

If you are using just one stick or crutch, always use it on the opposite side to where the pain is e.g. if it's your left knee that is sore, hold the stick in your right hand. The reason for this is that when we walk normally we swing our opposite arm with our opposite leg (think of the army marching). This is the most efficient way for our body to move, so we want to mimic that when using a walking aid. You can find out more about how to use crutches safely and effectively, including how to get up and down stairs with them in Chapter 17.

9) Knee Braces

Braces can be worn to help stabilise the leg and reduce the pressure going through the joint. They are really good if the knee is feeling weak and wobbly. There are lots of different types of arthritis braces available. The most high-tech ones redistribute forces away from the part of the knee affected by the arthritis, which can dramatically reduce pain. Others provide more general support.

10) Footwear

If you are suffering from arthritis knee pain, wear shoes with low heels and soft cushioned soles. High heeled shoes change the way the forces act on the knee putting increased pressure on the knee joint, so avoid! Cushioned soles will help reduce the forces going through the knee by acting as shock absorbers. Insoles can be helpful if you have problems with your foot arches - having flat feet increases the pressure through the inner side of the knee. Foot position can often be corrected by wearing specially designed insoles in your shoes. If you think there may be a problem with your foot position, see an Orthotist or Podiatrist.

11) Acupuncture

There have been a number of studies which show that acupuncture can help reduce pain and disability with knee arthritis[12]. Acupuncture works by blocking pain signals, releasing endorphins and increasing blood flow to the area. It should only ever be carried out by a qualified professional, and isn't suitable for everyone. People often find that the benefits of acupuncture build up over time.

12) Surgery

Many people will be able to manage their arthritis using the treatment options we have just talked about, but for some, the pain and disability may progress to the point when surgery is required. The most common surgery performed for knee arthritis is a knee replacement, where the damaged part of the joint is removed and replaced with an implant. We will look at this in much more detail in the second-half of this book.

Chapter 6: Alternative Medicine

Alternative medicine is becoming increasing popular for the treatment of arthritis. There is more and more research being done into the effectiveness of different types of alternative treatment and many people swear by them.

The Arthritis Foundation reports that approximately sixty percent of arthritis sufferers have tried alternative home remedies for arthritis. People are generally looking for help relieving things like pain, stiffness, depression, anxiety, stress and poor sleep that often accompany arthritis.

Some natural arthritis remedies can work really well and more research is being done to look into their effectiveness. However, many more don't work or haven't been studied enough to produce sufficient evidence.

We are going to look at supplements, homeopathy and other home remedies that may help, but before we start:

SAFETY ADVICE: Never turn down proven conventional therapy in favour of natural arthritis relief. Always check with your doctor before taking any natural remedy, especially if you are on any medication. Herbal supplements can have strong side effects and they could have unknown and potentially dangerous interactions with medication. Prescribed drugs are very carefully regulated and checked for side effects. Herbal drugs do not have to go through any safety tests before going on the market, so do be aware. Some studies have shown that what is on the label doesn't always match what is on the bottle of natural herbal remedies so use caution and always buy them from a reputable retailer.

1) Supplements

Supplements are one of the most popular types of natural remedies for arthritis. Here are some of the most popular ones:

Omega-3 Fatty Acids: Omega-3 fatty acids found in fish are thought to reduce inflammation[13]

Glucosamine: Glucosamine is a naturally occurring substance found in joints and connective tissue. Its main functions are to repair cartilage and maintain joint mobility and manufacturers claim it slows the deterioration of cartilage[14]

Chondroitin: Manufacturers claim chondroitin reduces pain and inflammation, improves joint function and slows the progression of arthritis[15]

SAM-e: SAM-e is a natural chemical found in the body that supposedly increases blood levels of proteoglycans - molecules that seem to play a key role in preserving cartilage by helping to keep it plumped up and well oxygenated[16]

Should I Try Supplements?

Any natural remedy that does provide relief tends to work to reduce symptoms, rather than stopping the progression of the disease. Many supplements, whilst having little research behind them, also have very few side effects, so whilst the scientific evidence may not be there, they may be worth a try. Usually there is no harm in trying supplements, but this is not always the case – some can have side effects.

2) Homeopathy

Homeopathy has been used for centuries and involves using natural products to help reduce arthritis pain, inflammation and stiffness without the need for man-made chemicals. It takes very small doses from plants and/or minerals and uses them to boost the body's immune system.

Scientifically, the research behind homeopathy is mixed, but more and more arthritis patients are turning to it to relieve persistent symptoms. Let's look at four of the best.

Avocado Soybean Unsaponifiables (ASU): It claims to slow arthritis progression and reduce pain by reducing inflammation. A study in 2003 by the Journal of Rheumatology reported that ASU inhibited the breakdown of cartilage and promoted repair[17].

Boswellia: aka Indian Frankincense is thought to be a powerful anti-inflammatory and painkiller. It may also prevent cartilage loss. In one study, it decreased arthritis pain by over 80%. In another study, people taking Boswellia reported less pain, better mobility and were able to walk further than those taking a placebo pill[18]

Feverfew: It is thought that Feverfew reduces the production of substances that cause and prolong inflammation. Some studies have found that the anti-inflammatory effects of this herb are greater than those achieved by NSAIDs (non-steroidal anti-inflammatories e.g. ibuprofen)[19].

Ginger: It is thought that Ginger works by increasing circulation which takes inflammatory chemicals away from arthritic joints. Studies have shown its results to be similar to anti-inflammatories such as ibuprofen and Celebrex, and that it reduces pain with standing and walking in OA sufferers[20].

Other homeopathy options that may help with arthritis include Evening Primrose Oil, Thunder God Vine, Willow Bark, Cherries, Dandelion Leaves and Celery.

Should I Try Homeopathy?

Homeopathy uses extremely small doses of natural products and therefore often has fewer side effects than conventional medicines. However, this is not always the case. Some homeopathy products can have serious side effects, and may interact adversely with other drugs with potentially serious side effects. You should always consult your doctor and a professional homeopath before taking any homeopathy products. Whilst the scientific evidence behind arthritis homeopathy products is often lacking, some people do find considerable benefit from using them. It can take up to a couple of months to notice the effects from homeopathic substances.

3) Other Home Remedies

Here are some other simple home remedies you might want to try:

Anti-inflammatory Gel/Cream: such as Ibuprofen gel is a non-steroidal anti-inflammatory cream that is rubbed into the affected area to reduce pain and inflammation. It works locally at the site of application rather than systemically through the whole body like tablets so has less side effects

Capsaicin Cream: Capsaicin is the substance that gives peppers their "heat". By rubbing on capsaicin cream you irritate nerve endings which diverts your brains attention away from pain, reducing pain levels[21]

TENS Machine: A TENS machine (transcutaneous electric nerve stimulation machine) involves placing electrode pads around a joint which deliver small electric pulses to the area. TENS works by suppressing pain signals to the brain and encouraging the body to produce higher levels of endorphins, the body's natural painkillers. While TENS is a very safe way to treat pain, care must be taken with where the pads are placed. TENS tends to provide short term pain relief and can help to reduce stiffness

Magnets: Magnets are a popular alternative medicine for arthritis. Manufacturers claim they reduce pain and inflammation, increase blood flow and promote general well-being and relaxation. However, the claims are as yet unproven scientifically. That said, some people swear by them. One of the best ways to get the benefits of magnetic therapy is to wear a magnetic knee brace where the magnets surround the joint.

Copper Bracelets: Wearing copper bracelets is another popular alternative treatment for arthritis. One study in Australia compared the use of aspirin and aspirin coupled with copper magnets in the treatment of arthritis. The results showed the group using the copper bracelets responded better than the group using aspirin in isolation[22]. Some copper bracelets also have magnets in them for added benefit.

Climate: Many people find that a cold, damp climate aggravates their symptoms and find that going to warm climates during winter can help to reduce their pain. Arthritis sufferers often comment that they know when bad weather is coming because their joints start hurting. One theory is that it is the change in air pressure that affects symptoms.

Should I Try Them?

Whilst the scientific evidence is often lacking when it comes to alternative medicine for arthritis, that doesn't mean it should be ignored. Lots of arthritis sufferers report finding them a great addition to more conventional treatment. However, please remember you should never opt for alternative medicine over proven conventional treatments. They should be used as an adjunct, not a replacement. And you should always check with your doctor for using any form of alternative medicine to check it is safe for you.

Chapter 7: Diet And Arthritis

Food choices can make a real difference to your quality of life. By making simple changes to your diet and knowing which foods to eat and which to avoid with arthritis, you can reduce pain and inflammation. Whilst you cannot cure arthritis by following a particular diet, making good food choices can have a big impact.

The main considerations to be aware of are that you are aiming to reduce inflammation and ensure a healthy body weight. These will help to reduce the stress and irritation of the affected joints. So when thinking about the best diet for arthritis, it is important to be aiming for a healthy, balanced diet combined with a healthy lifestyle and regular exercise. If you are thinking of changing your diet, always discuss this with your doctor or dietician first.

Foods To Avoid With Arthritis

1) Fried Food: the reason to avoid fried food (such as French fries, fried chicken, donuts) with arthritis is two-fold. Firstly, when eaten in excess they increase body fat which places more stress through joints which can lead to wear and tear. Secondly, fried food is often cooked in hydrogenated oils, commonly known as Trans fats (see below)

2) Fats: Avoid foods that contain the bad fats. These fall in to 3 groups:

Saturated Fats: such as full fat dairy products (e.g. butter), processed foods (e.g. cakes), some vegetable oils (e.g. palm oil) and certain meats.

They can increase inflammation around the body as well as increase your cholesterol levels

Trans Fats: These are the worst kind of fat and whilst they are being used less frequently, they can sometime be found in processed food such as fried food, biscuits and sweets. Trans fats occur naturally in some dairy and meat products, but most is formed from an industrial process that makes oil more solid and increase the shelf life of food products. They can increase cholesterol levels which can lead to heart disease. They tend to be labelled "partially hydrogenated oil"

Polyunsaturated Fats: You may have heard that Omega-3 is a useful kind of fat found in things like oily fish, but omega-6 polyunsaturated fat from things like corn, sunflower or vegetable oil increases inflammation. It is often found in baked goods, ready-made frosting and fried foods.

3) AGE's (Advanced Glycation End Product): These tend to be found in processed food or foods cooked at high temps like BBQ or fried food. Consuming excessive AGE's increases you risk of inflammation and developing type 2 diabetes. You can reduce AGE consumption by changing your cooking methods – lower the heat, opt for moist cooking (e.g. in a sauce) rather than dry cooking (e.g. grilling or skillet pan) or if you are dry cooking, add some lemon juice or vinegar as the acidity reduces AGE levels.

4) Sugars: Anything with high sugar levels e.g. fruit juice, cakes, soft drinks and sweets/candy raises your blood-sugar levels which can cause an inflammatory reaction in your body flaring up arthritis. One can of soda contains more than the recommended daily allowance of 32g sugar.

5) Refined Carbohydrates: Another food to avoid is anything made from refined carbohydrates such as white flour (plain or self-raising) or white rice. When white flour is made, the bran and germ parts are removed and they are the healthiest parts. Refined carbohydrates also increase cytokine levels and other inflammatory compounds which aggravate arthritis. Switch instead to wholegrain rice, bread and cereals

6) Alcohol: has been linked to flare ups in different types of arthritis, particularly gout. The worst culprits are beer, stout and fortified wines

7) Salt/Sodium: Most people consume much more salt each day than the recommended amount of less than 2,300mg. High levels of sodium are often found in processed food and can cause high blood pressure. Studies have recently found a link between high salt intake and auto-immune response, where the body produces inflammatory cells and starts attacking itself such as rheumatoid arthritis and ankylosing spondylitis (arthritis of the spine)

8) Large Portions: As we get older, we need smaller portions to maintain our weight and energy levels so we need to adjust how much we put on our plate to ensure we aren't over eating

9) Red Meat: some studies have shown a link between eating lots of red meat and inflammatory arthritis. Red meat tends to be fattier and the fats are easily turned into pro-inflammatory chemicals

10) Smoking: Not technically food or drink but tobacco has been linked with an increased risk of developing rheumatoid arthritis

Other thoughts on foods to avoid often include citrus fruits such as lemons and grapefruit and certain vegetables such as potatoes, peppers, chillies and tomatoes. However there is no scientific fact behind this and they are actually rich in anti-oxidants which can help slow arthritis progression.

If you think that a certain food is aggravating your arthritis, the best way to check is a dietary "exclusion and challenge". Cut the food type out of your diet for one month then gradually reintroduce it. If your symptoms flare up in the next few days, it is likely that the food is a trigger. It is always best to discuss allergies and irritants with a dietician before deciding what food to avoid to make sure you aren't losing out on vital vitamins and minerals.

Arthritis Food That Can Help

As well as there being food to avoid with arthritis, there are things that you can eat which may help.

1) Healthy Balanced Diet

It is really important to ensure you are getting a healthy, balanced diet when choosing arthritis food. The US Food & Drug Administration recommends ensuring you are having some of all the different food groups but splitting up your diet so it is:

Two Thirds: Fruit and vegetables (particularly colourful ones as they are high in antioxidants) and whole grains e.g. brown rice and oatmeal

One Third: Fat-free or low-fat dairy (e.g. skimmed milk) and lean protein (chicken, seafood, beans, nuts, seeds)

Fascinating Fact! Did you know, skimmed and semi-skimmed milk contains more calcium than full fat milk[23]

2) Omega-3 Rich Foods

Omega-3 can help reduce inflammation in two ways by inhibiting enzymes that trigger inflammation and decreasing the synthesis of inflammation-spreading chemicals such as cytokines. Good sources of omega-3 include oily fish e.g. salmon and sardines, walnuts, linseed, pumpkin seeds, soy beans and rapeseed (canola) oil.

Top Tips

Best vegetables: leafy green vegetables e.g. spinach, broccoli, sweet potato, squash, carrots, dried beans and peas

Best meats: seafood and fish – especially oily fish for omega-3

Best snack: popcorn

Chapter 8: Arthritis Exercise Programme

As seen in earlier chapters, exercises are one of THE BEST treatments for knee arthritis. It is not as simple as saying do this one exercise and your knee will get better, but if you do a combination of strengthening, stretching and balance exercises, you should, after a few weeks, really notice the difference in your knee.

Here I will share with you some of the exercises that in my experience have been most beneficial to people with arthritis. Obviously, everyone is coming to this from different situations. The best exercises for you will depend on a number of factors such as the strength and mobility you already have, your fitness levels, pain levels and the stage of your arthritis. The best thing to do is to see a physical therapist who can assess your knee and identify your areas of weakness, tightness, stiffness and any biomechanical issues.

Here, I have grouped exercises according to the position that you do them in. In each group, they are ordered according to how challenging they are, starting with the easiest first. In no way am I expecting you to do all of the exercises here, pick the ones that feel best for you. Aim for two or three from each section initially. For each exercise I will explain the purpose of the exercise, how to perform it, how many repetitions to aim for and top tips on how to vary the exercise to make it easier or harder (when appropriate). The progressions should only be used once you can easily do the full number of repetitions of an exercise. Then in the next section, you will find a daily programme guide that you can follow if you wish.

1) Lying Down Exercises

These are great exercises to do in the mornings before you get up. They will help to loosen up your knee and get it going for the day and are a great way to combat that early morning stiffness so often associated with arthritis. You should find those first few steps are easier when you get up after doing some of these.

a) Quad Clenches

Purpose: Quads strengthening and knee extension. Strengthens the Quads without moving the knee and encourages full straightening of the knee, which is often lost with arthritis. This one may seem too simple to be effective, but it really does help!

Starting position: Lying flat on your back or sitting up. Leg and knee straight

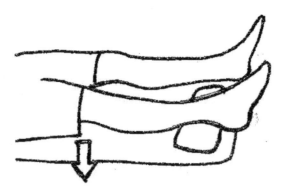

Action: Tighten the muscle on the front of the thigh by pushing your knee down into the bed, feeling your thigh clench. Hold for 3 seconds

Repetition: Repeat 10-30 times, 2-3x per day

Top Tips: If you are struggling to get your knee to straighten fully, place a rolled up towel underneath the ankle so that your leg is lifted slightly on the bed. Then do the exercise as described. Lifting the leg up slightly enables gravity to help the knee to straighten

b) Short Arcs

Purpose: Quads strengthening. Good strengthening exercise to start with, or one to do during flare ups as it doesn't require much knee movement

Starting Position: Lying flat on your back or sitting up with your leg horizontal on a flat surface such as a bed. Place a rolled up towel (approx. 10cm diameter) under the knee

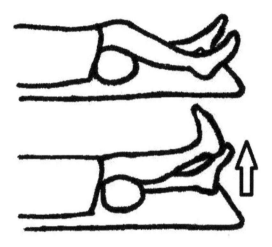

Action: Pull your toes towards you and clench your thigh muscles. Slowly lift your foot up off the bed until your knee is straight, keeping your knee resting on the towel. Hold for 3-5 seconds and slowly lower

Repetition: repeat 10-30 times, 2-3x daily

Progression: 1) Increase the size of the towel under the knee 2) Use a foot weight e.g. ankle weight or shoe

c) Heel Slides

Purpose: Movement and flexibility. One of the simplest yet most effective exercise to do first thing in the morning to loosen your knee up before you get up

Starting Position: Lying flat on your back or sitting up. Leg and knee straight out on the bed or along the floor.

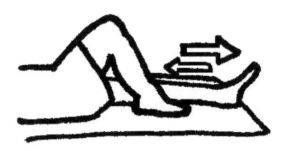

Action: Slide your heel towards your bottom as far as you comfortably can, bending your hip and knee. Keep your heel on the bed/floor. Hold for 3-5 secs and slowly return to starting position

Repetition: Repeat 10-30 times, twice a day. Gradually aim to bend your knee a little more each time

Progression: Carry out the exercise as above but when you've bent your knee as much as you can hook a towel over the ankle and pull it towards you to help the knee bend further – you can achieve the same effect by hooking your opposite foot over the ankle and gently pushing with that leg to increase the knee bend

Top Tip: Place a smooth board or a plastic bag underneath your foot so you have a slippery surface making it easier to move

d) The Shoulder Bridge

Purpose: Strengthening. Excellent strengthening exercise for the hamstrings, quads and buttock muscles

Starting Position: Lie on your back with both knees bent about 90° and your feet on the floor/bed

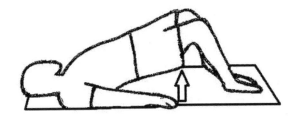

Action: Clench your buttocks and lift your bottom off the bed as high as you can without arching your back. Hold for 3-5 seconds and slowly lower

Repetition: Repeat 10-25 times, 1-2x daily

Top Tips: 1) Keep your back straight – don't let it arch as you lift up, it should be your bottom doing the work 2) don't hold your breath – keep breathing normally

e) The Clam

Purpose: Strengthening. This one is a must. A lot of people with arthritis have weak glutes (buttock muscles). This changes the way the forces go through the knee placing extra weight through the joint, especially the medial (inner) side. This can be reduced by strengthening the glutes

Starting Position: Lie on your side with your feet together, hips slightly bent and knees bent approximately 90°

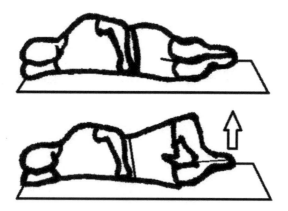

Action: Keeping your feet together, lift the top knee up as high as you can. Hold for 3 seconds and slowly lower

Repetition: Repeat 10-25 times on each side, 2x daily

Top Tips: The exercise gets its name as the movement is like that of a clam shell opening. Keep the feet together (toes and heels) and make sure the hips stay forwards, don't let them roll back

Progression: 1) Clench your buttocks together at the top of the movement to work them harder 2) Change the starting position slightly by lifting both feet up to hip height and opening up from there (still keeping the heels together). The greater range makes the muscles work harder 3) Squeeze your heels together as you do the exercises to work your glutes even harder

2) Seated Exercises

These exercises are great to do any time you are sitting in your chair for more than about half an hour to stop the knee from seizing up.

a) Hamstrings Clenches

Purpose: Strengthening. Strengthen the hamstrings muscles without having to move the knee

Starting Position: Sit in a chair with your heel against the leg of the chair

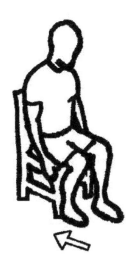

Action: Press your heel firmly backwards into the chair leg feeling the back of your knee and thigh tightening/clenching. Hold for 3-5 secs

Repetition: Do 10-20 repetitions, 2-3x daily

Top Tips: The foot and leg shouldn't move during this exercise, you should just feel the muscles tightening. Keep the rest of your body relaxed. You can also do this exercise in lying with your knee very slightly bent, by pushing your heel down into the bed

b) Buttock Clenches

Purpose: Strengthening. Strengthen the Glutes without having to move the knee

Starting position: Sitting up.

Action: Clench your buttocks together and hold for 3 seconds. You should feel yourself rise up slightly

Repetition: Repeat 10-20 times, 2-3x daily

Top Tip: You could also do this exercise lying down if you prefer

NB No picture for this one as it's pretty self-explanatory!

c) Leg Arcs

Purpose: Strengthening & mobility. A must any time you are sitting down for more than twenty minutes as it prevents stiffness setting in and the associated discomfort on first standing up. It helps increase mobility in the knee and also strengthens the knee at the same time

Starting position: Sitting on a firm chair with your knee bent and your foot on the floor.

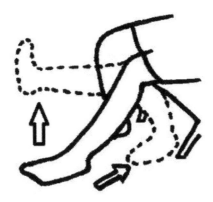

Action: Lift your foot up and straighten your knee as much as possible. Hold for 3-5 secs and slowly lower your leg down to the floor. Then slide your foot back as far as you can, hold for 3-5 seconds and return to starting position. Do all this in one fluid motion.

Repeat: 10-25 times, regularly during the day

Top Tip: It may help to have a towel or plastic bag under your foot to reduce the friction when sliding your foot backwards

Progression: *1) To improve strength:* Strengthen further by adding a weight either by wearing a shoe or ankle weights *2) To improve flexion* a) Hook your other foot around the front of the ankle and gently push backwards with it to further bend your knee b) Once you have slid your heel back as far as you can, lift your bottom up slightly using your arms and slide forwards keeping your foot still. You will find this makes your knee bend even more

d) Ankle Spins

Purpose: Mobility. The knee needs to be able to twist to move properly and this rotation movement is often one of the first things lost with arthritis. Regain it with this exercise

Starting Position: Sit in a firm chair, feet approximately 6 inches apart. If possible, have your knees together

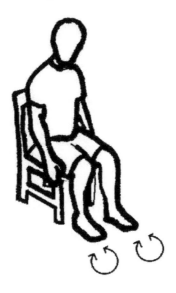

Action: Turn your feet inwards as far as you can and then outwards

Repetition: Spend a few minutes doing this twice a day

Top Tip: Ideally, you want to keep your knees together with this exercise to ensure the rotation is coming from your knee rather than your hip. If this is not possible, you can do it with your knees apart, but try and isolate the movement to your knee, not your hip and thigh.

e) Sit to Stand

Purpose: Strengthening, mobility & function. This is a great arthritis exercise as it works lots of muscles at the same time (quads, hamstrings and glutes), and is also very functional – it's a movement we do frequently during the day, but normally only once at a time.

Starting position: Sit in a firm chair, feet on the floor

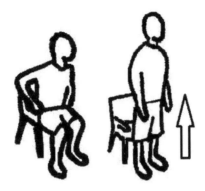

Action: Lean forwards, lift your bottom and stand up straight and then sit back down

Repetition: Repeat 10-30 times

Top Tips: You can make this exercise easier by 1) Pushing up through your arms too 2) Using a higher chair

Progression: 1) Don't push through your arms 2) Use a lower chair 3) Increase the speed you do the exercise - time yourself to see how many you can do in 1 minute and retest every few days to see what progress you are making 4) Hold a heavy weight – e.g. bag of books while you do the exercise

3) Standing Exercises

When you first start doing these exercises, make sure you hold onto something stable like a counter top, the wall or a chair. As you progress you may be able to stop holding on to help improve your balance as well as your strength

a) Kick Backs

Purpose: Strengthening & mobility. This a good exercise for the early stages of rehab. It helps strengthen the knee, targeting the hamstrings and also helps improve flexibility

Starting Position: Stand up straight holding on to something stable e.g. chair or table

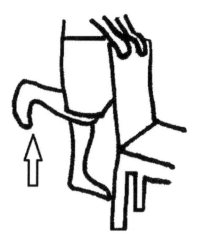

Action: Lift your foot up as far as you can towards your bottom, bending the knee. Hold for 3-5 secs

Repetition: Repeat 5-25 times, 2x daily

Progression: Add a weight e.g. shoe or ankle weight

Top Tips: 1) Don't bend forwards - keep your body upright 2) Don't let your thigh come forwards, keep your knees in line with each other

b) Knee Dips

Purpose: Strengthening. These mini squats strengthen the quads and get the knee moving

Starting Position: Standing, feet hip distance apart, toes pointing forwards. Hold onto something stable the first few times you do these for balance if needed

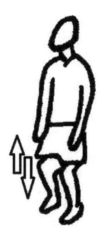

Action: Bend the knees slightly, taking your bottom backwards as if you were going to sit back on a chair. Then come back up to the starting position

Repetitions: Repeat 10-30 times 2x daily

Top Tips: 1) The knee should bend in line with the 2nd toe, not dropping inwards over the big toe 2) Make sure your knees don't come forwards as you squat – if you look down you should be able to see your toes

Progression: For more of a challenge try doing this exercise standing on one leg

PLEASE NOTE: The rest of these standing exercises are more challenging, so make sure you can confidently do the standing and lying exercises first.

c) Step Ups

Purpose: Strengthening & function. This is a great strengthening exercise that also helps reduce knee pain on stairs

Starting Position: Stand facing the bottom of the stairs or a single step. Hold onto the wall/rail for support if required

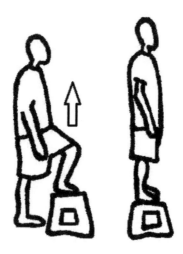

Action: Step up onto the first stair, one foot at a time, leading with the leg you want to strengthen. Without turning round, step both feet back down in the opposite order (i.e. to strengthen the right leg, lead with the right on the way up and the left on the way down)

Repetition: Repeat 10-30 times, 2x daily

Progression: 1) Don't hold onto anything 2) Keep the leg to be worked up on the step and just move the other leg up and down

Top Tip: If you don't have any steps at home, be creative e.g. telephone directory

d) Step Downs

Purpose: Strengthening, balance & stability. Another great all-rounder - strengthens the knee, improves balance and knee stability

Starting Position: Stand sideways on top of a step. Hold the wall/rail for support

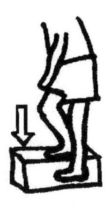

Action: Slowly lower one leg down to the floor and then bring it back up (keeping your other foot up on the step throughout). You will be working the leg that stays on the top step, rather than the one you lower

Repetition: Repeat 10-30 times, 2x daily

Progression: Stand facing forwards and step down instead of sideways, lightly touching the foot to the floor. Again, you will be working the leg that remains on the step rather than the one stepping down

Top Tips: 1) You are aiming to do this in a slow, controlled fashion 2) Don't let the knee twist inwards as it bends, keep it in line with your second toe so you can always see your big toe 3) Keep up tall – don't bend forwards 4) Try and skim the floor gently rather than putting all your weight down through the foot

e) Wall Squats

Purpose: Strengthening & control. A great twist on traditional squats. This version of squats strengthens the quads but stops too much weight going through the knee. One of my all-time favourite knee strengthening exercises. This is a good one to do once you can happily do the knee dips

Starting position: Stand with your back against the wall, feet shoulder width apart a few inches away from the wall, toes pointing forwards

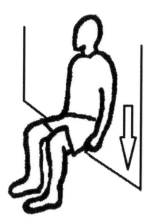

Action: Slowly slide down the wall a few inches bending your knees. Hold for 3-5 seconds and slowly push up to starting position.

Repetition: Repeat 10-25 times, 2x daily

Progression: 1) Increase the depth of the dip 2) Hold the bent knee position for longer (aiming for 10secs)

Top Tips: 1) As you squat, don't let your knees come too far in or out - keep your knee in line with your second toe so you can always see your big toe past the inside of your knee 2) If there is too much friction from the wall, try doing it against a closed door or with a plastic bag behind your back

f) Single Leg Standing

Purpose: Improve balance. Balance is often affected with arthritis. As a quick test to see whether you would benefit from balance exercises, try standing on one leg with your eyes closed. If you can't do it for one minute, you would benefit from this exercise as it helps your body learn the subtle adjustments needed for good balance.

Starting position: Standing

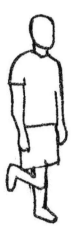

Action: Lift up your one foot and stand on one leg for as long as you can

Repetition: Spend five minutes doing this 2x daily

Progression: 1) Close your eyes 2) Throw and catch a ball – eyes open! 3) Slowly bend and straighten your knee a small amount (eyes open initially and then closed)

Top Tips: Get into the habit of practising this during the day e.g. when brushing your teeth or waiting for the kettle to boil

Planning A Daily Exercise Programme

Ideally, arthritis knee exercises should be done at least five times per week. You don't need to do all of the exercises, pick the ones that feel best for you.

Here you will find a daily exercise plan that means you split the exercises into sets rather than having to do them all at the same time. This way, each set will take you less than five minutes, making it much more manageable to fit into busy days.

This programme gives you a mix of strengthening, movement and balance exercises. I have grouped them into four sets. In each set there are two stages, stage 1 are the easier exercises that anyone should be able to perform, and stage 2 are more challenging. Please make sure you can confidently do the stage 1 exercises before progressing on to stage 2, and remember, some will be easier than others so you might want to do a mixture of stage 1 and stage 2 exercises for a while.

Please tailor this to suit you – some exercises may be too easy or too difficult for you initially and therefore not appropriate. It really depends what stage your arthritis is at. Find what works best for you - the people who have the most success are those who stick with their exercise programmes.

Set 1: Morning (Before Getting Out of Bed)

Stage 1: *Lying:* Quads Clenches, Short Arcs, Heel Slides and Buttock Clenches

Stage 2: *Lying:* Heel Slides, Shoulder Bridge, and The Clam

Set 2 & 3: Late Morning AND Afternoon

Stage 1: *Sitting:* Buttock Clenches, Hamstring clenches, Long Arcs, Ankle Spins. *Standing:* Kick Backs, Knee Dips, Sit to Stand

Stage 2: *Sitting:* Long Arcs. *Standing:* Step Ups, Step Downs, Wall Squats, Single Leg Standing

Set 4: Evening

Stage 1: *Lying:* Quad clenches, Short Arcs and Heel Slides

Stage 2: *Lying:* Heel slides, Shoulder Bridge and The Clam

Anytime sitting for more than 20 mins: Long Arcs and Ankle spins

You can either do four sessions of exercises each day, or if you would prefer to only do exercises twice a day, combine set 1 and 2 in the morning and set 3 and 4 in the evening.

Chapter 9: Surgical Options

For many people, the treatments we have been talking about will be enough to get their symptoms under control. However, for others, this may not be the case. As arthritis progresses to stage 3, advanced arthritis, there is a high chance that surgery may be required.

There are three types of surgery that can help treat knee arthritis

1) Knee Arthroscopy: Key-hole surgery where damaged parts of cartilage are removed, known as a meniscectomy. This is only really suitable with mild or moderate arthritis (stages 1 & 2)

2) Osteotomy: Where a small amount of diseased bone is removed. If the leg is deformed, it can be straightened.

3) Knee Replacement: Where part or all of the joint is removed and replaced with a prosthesis (implant) made of metal and plastic

Knee replacements are by far the most common and effective surgery performed for arthritis, so we are going to concentrate on those.

Chapter 10: Knee Replacement Surgery

Knee joint replacements are most commonly carried out to treat advanced osteoarthritis of the knee, stage 3. They involve replacing the worn and damaged part of the knee with a new joint (prosthesis) made of metal and plastic to reduce pain and improve function.

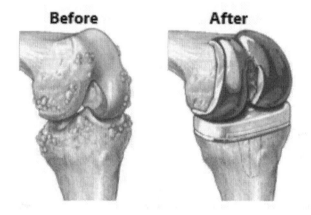

Knee replacements are the most common joint replacement surgery performed. Over 600,000 knee replacements are carried out each year in the US[24]. Knee replacements were first carried out in the 1940's and have developed significantly since then.

There are two types of knee replacement:

1) Partial Knee Replacement (PKR): where only one side of the joint is removed and replaced. It is sometimes known as a Unicompartmental Knee Replacement or Unicondylar Knee Arthroplasty.

This is only suitable when the arthritis is confined to one side of the joint, most commonly the medial (inner) side.

2) Total Knee Replacement (TKR): where the entire joint is replaced. It is also known as a Total Knee Arthroplasty. These are by far the most common with approximately 90% of knee replacements being total knee replacements[1]

We are going to look at both of these and see how they compare.

Total vs Partial Knee Replacement – Which Is Right For Me?

In the past, the whole knee had to be replaced, known as a total knee replacement (TKR) even if part of the knee joint was ok. But about thirty years ago partial knee replacement surgery was developed. It means it is possible to replace only one side of the knee joint so the unaffected part of the knee does not undergo unnecessary surgery which therefore leads to a quicker and fuller recovery.

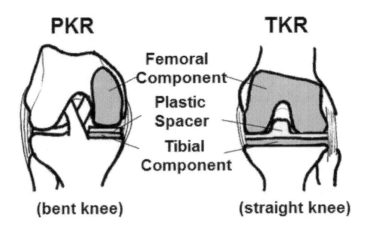

Now, if the arthritis is in both sides of your knee, you would need to have a total knee replacement. In one third of cases, knee arthritis only affects one side of the knee. It is six times more likely to be the inner (medial) side rather than the outer (lateral) which is affected.

Chapter 11: Knee Replacement Indicators

People are often unsure at what stage knee replacement surgery is appropriate. As we have already discussed, there is often little correlation between symptoms and x-ray findings with knee arthritis. There are no hard and fast rules but the following criteria are good guidelines that a knee replacement would be beneficial:

1) The pain is affecting your normal daily activities e.g. walking, stairs

2) The pain is affecting your sleep e.g. frequently keeps you awake or wakes you up

3) You have tried exercises to strengthen your knee for a reasonable period with no effect

4) You are in severe pain

If your symptoms are not as bad as these, surgery is usually not needed at the moment and other treatment methods are more appropriate.

Total or Partial Knee Replacement?

As well as the symptoms we have just discussed, there are strict criteria that assess for the suitability of a partial knee replacement over a total knee replacement. In order to have a partial knee replacement:

1) There can be no damage to the cartilage on the other side of the knee

2) There must be full thickness loss of cartilage on the affected side

3) Both cruciate ligaments (ACL and PCL) should preferably be intact (although this doesn't always have to be the case)

4) It is only suitable for osteoarthritis, not inflammatory arthritis

Some people worry about leaving it too long before having a knee replacement. Rest assured, there is no need to worry. Arthritis does not get to a stage where it is so bad that the surgery can't be performed, so there is generally no harm in waiting. However, if by waiting you are losing strength in your muscles from not being able to keep active, it is likely to take you longer to recover after surgery.

The Gender Effect

We like to think that the recommendation for surgery will be based on the correct combination of our symptoms (e.g. pain levels) and clinical findings (e.g. weakness and stiffness), but it may also be that gender plays a part. A Canadian study in 2008[25] looked at the effects of a patient's sex on the recommendation for total knee arthroplasty. 71 physicians (38 family physicians and 33 orthopedic surgeons) were asked to assess a male and female patient with identical symptoms and moderate arthritis on x-ray – the only difference between the subjects was gender. The study found that both sets of physicians were more likely to recommend a knee replacement to the male subject than to the female subject - the family physicians were 2 times more likely and the orthopaedic surgeons were 22 times more likely. This suggests that gender bias may contribute to the recommendation for surgery. Whilst this is most likely a largely unconscious bias, it may be worth seeking a second opinion if you feel you meet the criteria for a knee replacement but aren't being offered one.

10 Second Summary

Surgery is only advised when symptoms are severe and other treatments have failed. If the arthritis is on one side of the knee, you need a partial knee replacement, if it's on both sides, you need a total knee replacement.

Chapter 12: Preparing For Surgery

Whether it's a total or partial knee replacement, preparation for surgery will be similar. A few days or weeks before your surgery you will have a pre-op appointment where the surgeon will review your x-rays and talk you through what is going to happen. This is a good opportunity to ask any questions you may have. I always recommend writing your questions down before your appointment and taking the list with you, to make sure you don't miss anything. You may also want to make notes during your appointment to help you remember everything afterwards.

At the same appointment you should also see a physical therapist who will talk through the rehab and recovery process e.g. exercises for you to do after the operation. It is well worth doing these exercises for a few weeks before your surgery too as the stronger and more flexible your knee is before surgery, the quicker you will recover afterwards.

Knee replacement surgery (both total and partial) is usually carried out either by:

General Anaesthetic: you are put to sleep for the duration of the operation.

Spinal Anaesthetic: (epidural) which numbs the body below the waist. You are also given medicine to make you sleepy.

Chapter 13: What Happens In Surgery

Let's have a look at what actually happens during each type of operation.

Total Knee Replacement Surgery

A vertical incision (cut) is made on the front of the knee, usually about 20-25cms long. The kneecap is moved to the side to expose the joint. The surgeon removes the damaged bone and cartilage. The anterior cruciate ligament (ACL) is removed and often the posterior cruciate ligament (PCL) is too. The collateral ligaments at the side are preserved.

The bones are shaped to fit the new knee implant (prosthesis). Smooth, metal components are attached to the surfaces of the tibia and femur and held in place with cement, and a plastic insert sits between them. In some cases, the back surface of the patella may also be replaced with a plastic button if there is arthritis present there too. The wound is then sewn up with clip stitches. A dressing will be placed over the wound and the knee will then be bandaged to help reduce swelling.

Total knee replacement surgery takes about 2 hours.

Partial Knee Replacement Surgery

A smaller incision, around 12cms long, is made on the front of the knee to expose the joint and the surgeon will assess the joint to ensure that a partial knee replacement is suitable. The arthritic parts of the bones are removed with special saws and then replaced with the new joint (prosthesis) which is attached to the ends of the thigh and shin bones (femur and tibia) working to resurface the joint. The cruciate and collateral ligaments are preserved. The prosthesis is then secured in place with cement and the wound is stitched up, again with clips.

The operation takes about 1.5hrs.

Occasionally the extent of the arthritis does not show up clearly on x-ray and partial knee replacement surgery may not be suitable after all. If this is the case, the surgeon will perform a total knee replacement (TKR) instead. You should have been consented for this prior to surgery.

Chapter 14: What Happens After Surgery

After total or partial knee replacement surgery, you will return to your ward (after a short stay on the recovery ward) and the nurses will ensure you are getting adequate pain relief. You may have a small drain in your knee for the first 24-48 hours to remove any bleeding from the knee, and a drip in your arm to ensure you are receiving adequate fluids and medication.

Either later that day or the next morning, a physical therapist will come to see you and help you get out of bed. You will most likely be able to fully weight bear on your new knee (i.e. put as much weight through your leg as you feel comfortable doing) within 24 hours but you may need to use a frame, crutches or sticks for the first few days to help.

You will start your exercises straight away and will progress through the rehab programme as instructed by your physical therapist.

How Long Do You Stay In Hospital?

People are normally discharged from hospital after three to five days following a total knee replacement and one to two days following a partial knee replacement, depending on how they are doing.

Both the doctor and physical therapist will review you before discharge. Before you can go home, you should be able to:

1) Get in and out of bed by yourself

2) Walk safely with or without crutches/sticks/frame

3) Climb steps and stairs (unless you don't have any at home)

4) Fully straighten your knee

5) Bend your knee well, preferably at least 90° (it can take longer to achieve this if the movement was severely restricted prior to surgery)

Chapter 15: Knee Replacement Recovery

Most people make an excellent recovery after surgery and are up and about very quickly. Gone are the days when people were in hospital for two weeks or more. Now it's up and about straight away and home in just a few days. Recovery time will vary for each person, and may fluctuate, but here we will look at a general guide for what to expect.

Your knee will most likely be sore and swollen after your operation initially but often much less so than before the surgery as you will no longer be getting any arthritis pain. Your doctor will prescribe appropriate medication to be taken regularly to control pain and swelling, and in some cases to prevent infection.

For the first 7-10 days, you must keep the wound clean and dry until the stitches are removed. As the knee heals, the post-op pain will settle down, usually within a few weeks. You can help reduce the swelling by using ice and Tubigrip (a special compression bandage). When resting, it is advisable to have your leg elevated to help reduce swelling. Do make sure your knee is supported when elevating the leg, or else it will get stiff and sore.

After about a month you should notice quite a dramatic improvement in your knee. You can stop using any walking aids such as crutches or sticks as soon as you feel able – usually within a few days, and certainly by six weeks. You can return to driving after 4-6 weeks, as long as you can perform an emergency stop. It is always a good idea to check with your insurance company after your surgery, before you start driving again.

You will usually have a follow-up appointment with your surgeon after around 6 weeks to check your progress.

The majority of the pain and swelling should settle within around 3 months but you will continue to make improvement for up to 2 years after your operation.

Returning To Activities

For around 6-8 weeks after surgery you should avoid:

• Any pivoting (twisting) on your knee

• Kneeling

• Squatting

After 6-12 weeks, you should be able to return to most activities, such as swimming. You may need to make some slight modifications to certain activities e.g. golf – don't wear shoes with spikes, so that you don't over-twist your knee.

There are a few activities it is advisable to avoid completely after a total knee replacement as they place excessive stress through the joint. These include jogging, contact sports (e.g. basketball and football), squash, badminton, jumping activities and skiing. If you are unsure, discuss things with your doctor or physical therapist and check what is right for you.

Returning To Work

It will depend on the nature of your job as to when you can return to work. For example if you have a manual job or are on your feet for long periods it may take longer to return to work than if you have a more sedentary job. Your doctor will be able to advise you as to when it is safe to return.

Chapter 16: Goals

It's important to remember that we are all individuals and that the recovery process will be slightly different for each person. How quickly you recover will depend on a number of things, but here is a guide as to what goals you should be aiming for during the initial period of the recovery process. If you feel you aren't achieving these goals, talk to your surgeon or physical therapist.

Goals: Weeks 1-3

The main aims in the first few weeks focus on getting the pain and swelling under control and getting the knee moving again. You are aiming to:

1) Bend your knee at least 90 degrees (a right angle)
2) Get the knee almost fully straight (5 degrees of bend)

A good guide for this is to see how many fingers you can get underneath your knee when it is straight – you are aiming for three or less

Goals: Weeks 3-6

At this stage, you should be working on more challenging exercises to improve the movement of your knee as well as your strength, stability and balance. It should be feeling much easier to move around. You are aiming to:

1) Bend your knee between 105 and 120 degrees

2) Fully straighten your knee

3) Walk and go up and down stairs normally with no aids

Goals Weeks 6-12

By this stage, you should be feeling confident to start returning to some of your normal activities and you should be able to do more challenging exercises. You are aiming to:

1) Walk longer distances without a limp

2) Fully straighten your knee

3) Bend your knee between 105 and 120 degrees (or more!)

Measuring Progress

There is nothing more encouraging than seeing progress in those first few weeks, but it can sometimes be difficult to recognise what progress you are making. In the same way that other people notice children growing more than the children or their parents themselves do, you will probably find that it is the people around you who spot the progress you are making more than you.

Here are a couple of simple things you can be doing at home to keep track of what progress you are making in terms of regaining movement at your new knee.

Measuring Knee Bend

This is a great way to keep track of how much your knee is bending.

1) Place a chair near the wall so that when you sit down, your feet are flat and your toes are touching the wall

2) Gently slide your bottom forwards towards the front of the chair to bend your knee as much as feels comfortable

3) Measure the gap between the front of your knee and the wall.

Measure The Gap   **Goal**

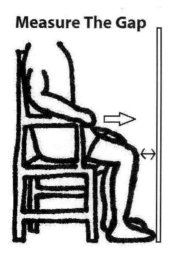 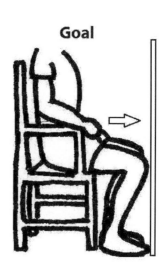

Make sure you use the same chair each time you do this test. Don't worry if your knee seems a long way from the wall to start with, remember that you are looking for progress.

Measuring Knee Extension

This one is a little trickier and you will need someone to help.

1) Lie on your back with your leg out straight

2) Keeping your foot relaxed, squash the back of your knee down towards the bed/floor by tightening your thigh

3) Get someone to measure the gap between the back of your knee and the bed/floor

Measure The Gap   **Goal**

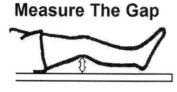 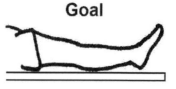

If you do these tests every few days, you should notice that the gaps get gradually less and less as your knee loosens up and bends and straightens more. People often find it easier to spot improvement in how much the knee bends than how much it straightens.

Chapter 17: Top Tips For Making A Great Recovery

Let me share with you my top tips on various activities in those first few weeks after surgery to help you get the best results. Everyone is different but these are the things I have seen work best over the years with my patients. Some of these can also be helpful for arthritis sufferers whether or not they need surgery, to make life easier.

1) Walking

The physical therapists will be along to help you get up within 24 hours of your surgery. You may initially need the support of a Zimmer frame or crutches, but by the time you go home you should have progressed to sticks or even no aid at all.

Walking is great exercise after a knee replacement both for your new knee, but also your whole body. Prolonged periods resting in bed or in a chair can lead to issues such as back pain, muscle weakness and stiffness. Start with short distances just around the home, but as the knee becomes more comfortable, try and get out of the house, gradually increasing the distance you walk. You are aiming to regain a completely normal walking pattern.

If you are using a walking aid e.g. a frame or crutches, use this movement sequence when walking:

a) Aid: place both crutches (or frame/sticks) about 12inches (1 foot) in front of you, slightly wider than hip distance apart

b) Operated Leg: Push down through the crutches and bring your operated "bad" leg forwards, level with the crutches

c) Unaffected Leg: Still pushing through the crutches, step the unaffected "good" leg forwards, initially level with the other foot, but as you progress, you will be able to bring this leg further forwards in front

Repeat this process using the mantra "aid, bad leg, good leg" over and over. This is known as a 3-point gait as there are three movements per stride. As you progress, you will be able to move the aid and the operated leg forwards together and then step through with the good leg, so you are back to the normal pattern of two movements per stride, rather than three.

d) Turning: Take little steps when you turn around, moving your crutches first so you don't twist your knee

The key things to aim for when you are walking are:

a) Technique: with each step aim to get the heel down first, transfer the weight forwards through the foot and finally push-off from your toes

b) Step Length: when we walk, we alternate putting one foot in front of the other. Aim to get the length of each step (distance between the front and back foot) equal on both sides.

c) Timing: try to spend the same length of time on each foot when you step – it is very easy to rush to get the weight off your operated leg as quickly as possible (a habit which may have formed before surgery due to your arthritis pain).

d) Speed: as your knee gets stronger and more flexible, try to gradually increase your walking pace back to your normal rhythm. Again, this may have slowed either prior to surgery due to arthritis pain, or from the initial pain after the operation. Everyone's natural walking speed (known as cadence) will vary slightly but the average number of steps taken per minute is around 100-120.

2) Getting In & Out of A Chair

Getting in and out of a chair sounds simple, but in the early days, especially if you are dealing with crutches (whether they are elbow crutches or axillary crutches that go under your arms), it can be a little tricky.

Best Way To Sit Down

a) Back up to the chair/bed/toilet until you can feel it on the back of your knees

b) If you are using elbow crutches, take your arms out of both arm loops and hold then in one hand on the side of your operated leg. You want to hold them together so the handles form an "H" shape. Never sit down with your arms still in the loops as you can damage your shoulders. If you are using axillary crutches, hold them in one hand with the handles together

c) Step your operated leg forwards slightly to prevent it bending too much when you sit

d) Reach back with your free hand for the arm rest

e) Slowly lower yourself down

f) Put your crutches/sticks down somewhere so you can easily reach them when you get up.

Best Way To Stand Up

This is basically the reverse!

a) Pick up your walking aids and hold them in one hand, on the side of your operation. ("H" shape for elbow crutches, handles together for axillary crutches)

b) Slide your operated leg out in front of you and shuffle forwards to the front of the chair

c) Lean forwards and push from the chair/bed up to standing and then slide your operated leg back level with the other leg

d) With elbow crutches place your forearms into the loops one at a time and then separate the crutches, or with axillary crutches place them under your arms

e) Stand for a few moments to make sure you feel balanced (you can get a bit of a head rush or feel slightly feint initially if you have been sitting for a while), and then off you go!

3) Stairs

You should be given the opportunity to practice going up and down stairs before you are discharged from hospital. It may seem like a simple thing to do, but stairs can often be a problem after a knee replacement, especially if you are using crutches or sticks. Initially, you will find it easiest to go up one step at a time i.e. both feet end up on the same step. The best order to use to minimise the weight going through the operated knee as well as the amount it has to bend is:

Going Up Stairs:

1) Unaffected "good" leg

2) Operated "bad" leg

3) Crutches/sticks (if you need them)

Going Down Stairs:

1) Crutches/sticks

2) Operated "bad" leg

3) Unaffected "good" leg

Physical therapists often use the mantra "good leg up to heaven, bad leg down to hell" to help people remember which leg leads. The crutches/stick always stay with the bad leg and the good leg is always on the higher step.

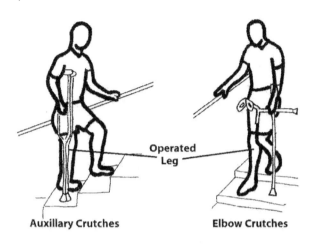

Auxillary Crutches   **Elbow Crutches**

If you have a bannister/hand rail, do use it as it provides more support. If you are using two sticks or crutches to walk, the easiest way is to hold the rail with one hand and hold the crutches in the other hand. If you are using elbow crutches or sticks, cross the spare crutch/stick into the other hand making a T-shape as shown in the diagram. Always hold the spare crutch on the outside of the "T" so if you do drop it, it doesn't bang against you and trip you up. If you are using axillary crutches, hold them together. Alternatively have a spare crutch/stick at the top of the stairs so you only have to carry one up - leave the other one at the bottom for when you come down.

Once you are no longer needing the crutches/sticks, initially stick to the same pattern of leading with your good leg on the way up and your bad leg on the way down one step at a time. In time you will be able to progress on to a reciprocal pattern where you only place one foot on each step.

4) Positions For Sleep/Rest

You will most likely be more tired than usual in the first few weeks following your operation. It is important that you get enough rest so the knee can heal. Here is some advice on the best positions to rest in:

In Bed

Side lying: if you want to lie on your side, it is best to lie on the un-operated side. Place a pillow under the operated leg to support the knee

Lying on your back: don't rest with a pillow/towel under the knee in bed if possible as this encourages the knee to stiffen in a slightly bent position – it is really important to regain full extension

Lying on your tummy: You may want to avoid this initially as it places pressure through the new knee and scar

In a Chair

Height: A higher chair will be easier to get in and out of

Position: keep the leg elevated to reduce swelling e.g. resting on a stool. Make sure the back of the knee is supported so it is not hanging down. However, make sure the knee is straight rather than bent to prevent stiffness and tightness setting in

Movement: Try to limit how long you sit for. Every 30 minutes or so, either get up for a little walk, or do your exercises in the chair to keep the knee moving.

5) Washing

Remember, you need to keep the wound and dressings dry until the stitches have been removed (usually around day 10). Those first few days you can wrap a plastic bag around the knee to help keep it dry when washing the rest of you, or initially stick to strip washes. After this, you should be able to bathe/shower normally, but always check with your doctor first. You may want to avoid the bath initially as it can be hard to get in and out unless you have a hand rail. One option is to get a bath seat that you can sit on in the bath to make it easier. Alternatively, use the shower, provided there isn't a large step up to get in. If you find it hard to stand for long, you can get a specially designed shower chair to sit on – don't use a normal dining chair or stool as they will slip!

Whether using the bath or shower, always take care as they can be very slippery and your knee muscles won't have regained all their strength yet. The last thing you want is to fall over. It is a good idea to make sure there is someone else in the house when you do bathe or shower initially, just in case you need some help.

6) Cars and Driving

It can be a little awkward initially getting in and out of the car. The best way is to open the door fully, turn so the seat is behind you and slowly lower yourself down into a sitting position (as described before). Then lift one leg in at a time.

Top Tips

a) Plastic Bag: put a plastic carrier bag on the seat to sit on – this makes it easier to swivel round in the seat as there is less friction

b) Put the seat back: as far as it will go, then you won't have to bend your knee so much

c) Use a high seat: If you can adjust the height of the seat, put it up as high as it goes – that way, you don't have to lower down quite so far and it makes getting out much easier. Alternatively, use a cushion or pillow to lift you a bit higher.

It normally takes around 4-6 weeks to return to driving. The pain needs to be under control, you need sufficient bend in the knee and must be able to perform an emergency stop. It is worth running through the movements required for an emergency stop procedure before you start the car. It is also a good idea to let your car insurance company know about your operation before driving.

7) Kneeling

It is important to avoid kneeling for the first six weeks, but after this, it is fine to try kneeling – you won't damage the new knee. It may well feel uncomfortable, in which case place a cushion or knee pad underneath. It is a good idea to check the surface you are going to be kneeling on for any debris as if there is numbness around the scar you may not notice if you a kneel on something sharp.

8) Preparing Your Home

It can really help to make a few changes at home before your operation to make things easier when you are discharged:

a) Rugs: remove any loose rugs or carpet as they are easy to trip on, especially with walking aids

b) Layout: move furniture around to ensure you will have enough space to move around, especially if you end up needing a frame or crutches initially

c) Bedroom: you may want to have a bed downstairs initially so you don't have to go up and down stairs, although in most cases this shouldn't be necessary

d) Simple Gadgets: Items such as a long handled shoe horn and grabbing tool can make things easier so you don't have to bend so much

e) Raised Toilet Seat: If your toilet is on the low side, you may want to get a raised toilet seat, a simple frame which sits over your toilet, so you don't have to lower down as far

f) Hand Rails: You may want to install some hand rails around the house e.g. up the stairs, in the bathroom, by any steps.

9) Medication

You will be given various medication to take home with you after surgery. These may include painkillers, blood thinners, anti-biotics and anti-nausea medication. If you were on any other medications prior to surgery, do check with your doctor as to whether it is safe to take them with the new medication. Take your medication as prescribed, and remember, it is much better to keep your pain under control with medication and be able to exercise than to try and struggle on without it.

10) Swelling

It is normal for there to be mild to moderate swelling for the first few months after a knee replacement. You can reduce this by:

a) Elevation: keep the leg elevated whenever possible (but remember to keep the knee straight)

b) Ice: Use ice packs regularly e.g. bag of frozen peas or gel ice pack wrapped in a towel and placed on the knee for 10 minutes at a time. Leave approximately 2 hours between applications. Remember the tips on ice safety that we discussed earlier

c) Compression Stockings: or Tubigrip compression bandage help to reduce swelling

If your knee swelling suddenly worsens, or you develop redness or oozing around your scar talk to your doctor immediately as it may be a sign of a blood clot or infection.

11) Exercise & Sports

Remember, sticking to your exercise programme is vital to making a full recovery. You will need to do exercises 2-4 times a day for at least 8 weeks. Don't stop until you have regained full strength and mobility in your new knee. Other things that can help are:

a) Walking: walking is great exercise. Aim to walk a little each day, gradually increasing as able, but remember, it is not a substitute for your knee exercises

b) Stationary Bike: cycling on a static bike is a great way to regain movement and strength in the knee. You may need to raise the height of the seat initially if you are having problems bending or straightening your knee

c) Swimming: swimming is a great way to exercise as it is low impact, but remember to wait until your stitches have been removed and the wound is dry

d) Low Impact: opt for low impact exercises e.g. cycling and golfing rather than high impact exercises such as running, skiing and squash

Remember, always check with your doctor or physical therapist before starting new activities to ensure your new knee is ready.

Chapter 18: The Rehab Process

Effective rehab is vital if you want to get the best results from your new knee. It doesn't matter if it is a total knee replacement or a partial knee replacement. When done correctly, rehab will help you regain movement, strength and balance, enabling you to get back to the activities you love, or even allow you to take up new ones.

Knee replacement rehab should start before you even have surgery. By doing exercises before surgery, you can improve the strength and flexibility of your knee. This helps with the recovery process for a number of reasons:

1) Better Support: for the new knee joint, making it easier to move around, with or without walking aids

2) Increases Confidence: you already know what to do so you can get going quicker

3) Good Habits: if you have gotten into the habit of doing exercises regularly before surgery, it is easier to keep going with them afterwards

4) Quicker Recovery: the more strength and movement you achieve before surgery, the easier it will be to maintain and improve both after surgery, even if things feel painful and tight to start with. You will be starting from a better place

Your physical therapist will show you a number of exercises to do to help regain the strength and movement in your knee. They will start with simple exercises that you can do lying down in bed and sitting in a chair and progress on to more advanced exercises to do in standing. We will look at some of the best exercises to do after surgery in the next chapter.

For the first few weeks, you will need to be doing exercises at least twice a day, every day, preferably three or four times a day. Over the weeks as the knee gets stronger and looser, your day to day activities will increase and you'll be able to cut down gradually on exercises.

You may need to continue with exercises for a few months - don't stop until you have regained full strength and full movement in your new knee, else there is a high risk of developing long term weakness, stiffness and pain.

How To Get The Best Results

One of the best predictors of outcome is a person's functional level and muscle strength prior to surgery. How much you stick to your rehab programme will have a big impact on the outcome of your knee replacement. If you exercise regularly before and after surgery, you should end up with a very strong, flexible knee that allows you to do almost anything you want.

If you don't exercise your knee you run the risk of developing long term stiffness and weakness in your knee which will limit function e.g. walking and climbing stairs. It is really important to be taking regular pain medication so you can start your rehab programme and get up and about. Always make sure you discuss this with your doctor. Follow their advice and don't worry that it is going to mask a problem in your knee. It will take the edge off the pain, but your knee will still let you know if you are doing something you shouldn't. Getting your knee moving again is one of the best ways to ensure you get the best results from your knee replacement.

Chapter 19: Knee Replacement Exercises

Your physical therapist will show you exercises to do, which may include some or all of the following. These exercises are intended as a guide – please always talk to your doctor or physical therapist before starting these exercises to ensure they are right for you. I have grouped them according to the position that they are carried out in. For each one, I will explain the purpose of each exercise (what it is going to achieve), how to perform the exercise, how often to do it and in some case variations to make the exercise easier or more challenging as you progress.

1) Lying Down Exercises

These exercises should be carried out on your bed, either lying down flat or sitting up with your leg stretched out straight.

a) Foot Pumps

Purpose: Promote good circulation in your leg and prevent Deep Vein Thrombosis (blood clot). This is one of the best exercises to start with after surgery

Action: Pull your foot up towards you, keeping the rest of your leg straight. Hold for 3 secs. Then point your toes down away from you. Hold for 3 secs

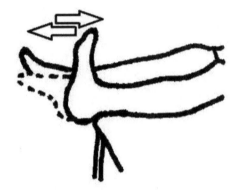

Repetition: Repeat for about 1 minute every 2-3 hours

Top Tip: You can stop doing this exercise once you are regularly walking around

b) Quad Clenches

Purpose: Maintain and strengthen the Quads without moving the knee, enable full straightening of the knee. This one almost looks too easy to be effective, but trust me, it is a great one to do!

Action: Tighten the muscle on the front of the thigh by pushing your knee down. You should feel your thigh muscles clench. Hold for 3 secs

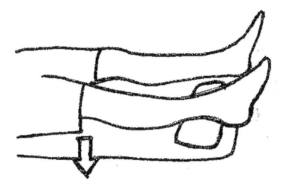

Repetition: Repeat 10-20 times every 3-4 hours

Variations: If you are struggling to get your knee to straighten fully, place a rolled up towel underneath the ankle so that your leg is lifted slightly on the bed. Then do the exercise as described. Lifting the knee up slightly lets gravity help the knee to straighten. However, don't rest in this position for more than a few minutes else the knee will get stiff and sore

c) Short Arcs

Purpose: Strengthen the Quads. Good exercise to start with as it doesn't require much knee movement. If you have a lag (the knee bends slightly when you try and lift the leg up straight), this one is a must!

Starting position: Place a rolled up towel (approx. 10cm diameter) under the knee.

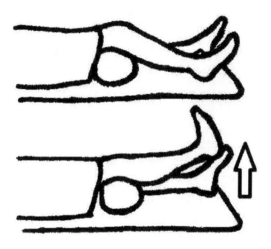

Action: Pull your toes towards you and clench your thigh muscles. Slowly lift your foot up off the bed until your knee is straight (keep your knee resting on the towel). Hold for 3-5 secs and slowly lower

Repetition: Repeat 10-30 times, 2-3x daily

Progression: 1) Increase the size of the towel under the knee 2) Add a weight e.g. by wearing a shoe, or using a light ankle weight. 3) Progress further by using a heavier weight (wait until you have good strength before doing this)

d) Straight Leg Raise

Purpose: Knee strengthening. Excellent exercise for strengthening the quads without having to bend the knee. Also makes getting in and out of bed easier NB Do not do this if you have a history of back problems

Action: Pull your toes towards you and tighten/clench the muscle on the front of the thigh, locking your knee straight (same action as with the Quads Clenches). Lift your foot up about 6 inches off the bed. Hold for 3-5 secs and slowly lower. Ensure your knee stays straight the whole time

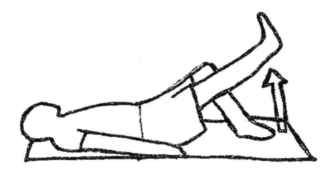

Repetition: repeat 10-20 times, 2x daily

Top Tip: You are aiming to lift the whole leg up straight without any lag (where the knee bends slightly before the foot comes up, due to weakness)

Progression: Add a weight e.g. by wearing a shoe, or using an ankle weight (again wait until you have good strength before doing this)

e) Heel Slides - Lying

Purpose: Regain knee flexion. This is really good exercise to do in the early stages to loosen your knee up without needing much strength

Action: Slide your heel towards your bottom as far as you comfortably can, bending your hip and knee. Keep your heel on the bed/floor. Hold for 3-5 secs and slowly return to the starting position

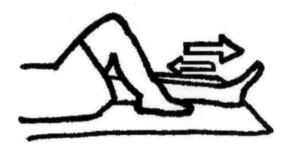

Repetition: Repeat 10-30 times, 2-3x daily. Gradually aim to bend your knee a little more each time

Variations: Make the exercise easier by placing a board and/or a plastic bag underneath your foot so you have a slippery surface making it easier to move

2) Seated Knee Replacement Exercises

You should be able to start these knee replacement exercises as soon as you are able to get out of bed. Sit in a firm, comfortable chair with your knee bent and feet flat on the floor to start.

a) Long Arcs

Purpose: Strengthen the quads and increase knee mobility. This one is great to do any time you are sitting for prolonged periods (30mins+) to stop the knee getting stiff

Action: Lift your foot up and straighten your knee as much as possible. Hold for 3-5 secs and slowly lower

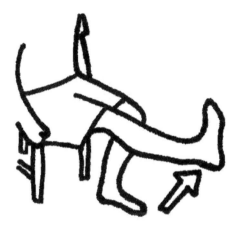

Repetition: 5-20 times, 3x daily

Progression: Strengthen further by adding a weight either by wearing a shoe or ankle weights

b) Seated Heel Slides

Purpose: Increase knee mobility and aid circulation. It seems very simple but is a great way to increase your range

Action: Slide your foot backwards on the floor as far as comfortable so you are bending the knee more. Hold for 3-5 secs

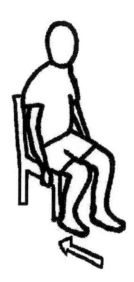

Repetition: Repeat 10-25 times, 3x daily

Progressions: 1) Hook your other foot around the front of the ankle and gently push backwards with it to further bend your knee. 2) Once you have slid your heel back as far as you can, keeping your foot still, raise yourself up on your chair using your arms and slide you bottom forwards keeping your foot still. You will find this makes your knee bend even more.

c) Knee Marching

Purpose: Three exercises in one - strengthens the quads and hip muscles, improves circulation and loosens up the legs when you've been sitting for a while.

Action: March your legs up and down one at a time. Lifting your knee and foot up and then back down

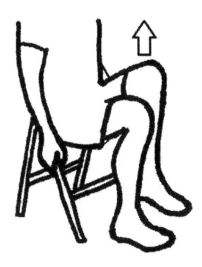

Repetition: Repeat for about 1 minute, twice a day and any time you are sitting for more than 20 mins to stop your knee getting stiff

Top Tips: As you get stronger, increase the speed you do this

d) Sit to Stand

Purpose: Improves knee mobility, strengthen and general fitness. This is a great exercise as it works lots of muscles at the same time (quads, hams and glutes), and is also very functional – it's a movement we do frequently during the day, but normally only once at a time.

Action: Lean forwards, lift your bottom and stand up straight and then sit back down

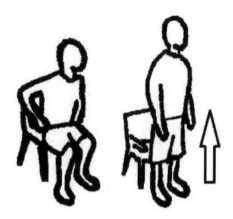

Repetition: Repeat 10-30 times

Top Tips: You can make this exercise easier by 1) Pushing up through your arms too 2) The higher the chair, the easier the exercise 3) If you are having problems bending your knee, put the foot slightly further forwards before doing this exercise

Progression: 1) Don't use your arms 2) Use a lower chair 3) Increase the speed you do the exercise at 4) Hold a heavy weight – e.g. bag of books while you do the exercise

3) Standing Knee Replacement Exercises

Once you are feeling confident on your feet, you can start these standing knee replacement exercises. For each one, stand with your feet slightly apart, weight equally distributed, holding onto something solid for balance.

a) Side Glides

Purpose: This helps you regain your confidence taking weight on your operated leg. There is often the tendency to favour the operated leg but it is really important to get back to taking full weight on your new knee as soon as possible otherwise you will likely walk with a limp

Action: Slowly shift your body weight over to one side. Hold this position for a few moments and then shift to the other side.

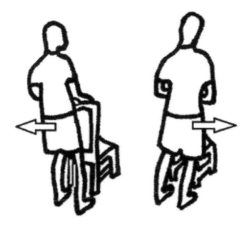

Repetition: Spend 3 or 4 minutes doing this twice a day

Progression: Aim to 1) increase how much weight you take on your operated leg 2) increase how long you keep your weight over on that side for 3) When you feel confident enough, let go of the chair as you do the exercise to help improve your balance

b) Kick Backs

Purpose: This helps strengthen the knee, targeting the hamstrings and also helps improve flexibility – both vital components of knee replacement rehab

Action: Lift your foot backwards as far as you can towards your bottom, bending the knee. Hold for 3-5 secs

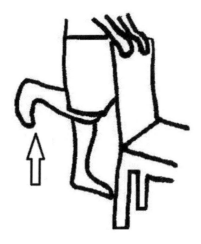

Repetition: Repeat 5-25 times, 2x daily

Top Tips: 1) Don't bend forwards - keep your body upright 2) try to keep your knees in line with each other- don't let your thigh come forwards

Progression: Add a weight e.g. shoe or ankle weight

c) Heel Raises

Purpose: Strengthen the calf muscles to help support the knee

Action: Rise up onto your toes lifting your heels as high as possible. Keep your body upright (don't bend forwards). Hold for 3-5 secs and slowly lower

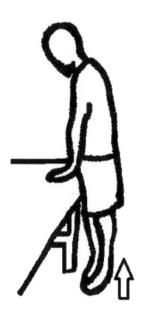

Repetition: Repeat 10-30 times, 2x daily

Top Tip: Once you can easily do 30 repetitions, try doing this exercise standing on one leg

d) Standing Marching

Purpose: Strengthen the quads, improve knee mobility and balance

Action: Lift one foot up off the floor, bending the knee and raising it towards the ceiling. Slowly lower down.

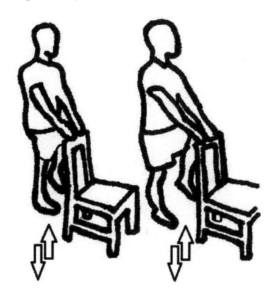

Repetition: 10-30 times, 2x daily on each leg

Top Tips: 1) Alternate which leg you are standing on - doing this exercise while standing on your operated leg helps improve balance and control, while lifting your operated leg improves strength and movement 2) Alternate the leg being lifted with each movement rather than doing it all on one side before swapping over

Chapter 20: What Exercises Are Right For Me?

It will really depend on what stage you are at and how the new knee is doing as to which are the best exercises for you. Ideally, to start with you want to be doing around five to six exercises at least three times a day. You want a combination of strengthening and movement exercises. Pick the ones that work best for you. It is really important that you are working at the right level for your knee. If you overdo things, your new knee won't thank you. But if you don't work it hard enough, you won't build up the much needed strength or mobility.

Working At The Right Level

Everyone recovers at a different speed following a knee replacement depending on factors such as age, fitness level, and the strength of each muscle. My advice is start slowly and gradually build up.

Follow the guidance of your physical therapist. Once you are home, initially carry on with the exercises you have been doing in hospital. When you feel ready to try a new exercise, start with a low number of repetitions on day 1, and stop — don't be tempted to do more. Sometimes, it can take a few hours for post exercise fatigue/discomfort to settle in. If the next day everything feels fine, next time increase the number of repetitions by 1 or 2. Then wait 24 hours and see how you feel. Carry on like this until you have reached the maximum number of reps recommended.

Here are some top tips on how to tell if you are working at the right level:

Not Working Hard Enough: If an exercise feels very easy to do and there are no ill-effects afterwards, you probably need to push things a bit more – either increase the reps, make the exercise more challenging e.g. with a weight, or move on to a different exercise instead

Getting it Just Right: As you do the exercises it should feel like you are working reasonably hard, but shouldn't be too painful. Any discomfort should stop within a few minutes of stopping the exercise.

Doing Too Much: If an exercise feels like really hard work, you are probably pushing things a bit too much. If you overdo things, your knee is likely to feel uncomfortable for a few hours after doing your exercises. If this happens, reduce the number of repetitions/weights

Re-evaluate regularly, aiming to progress your knee exercises approximately every three days.

The Next Stage

Once you can happily do all of these knee replacement exercises, which will probably take a few weeks, you can progress on to some of the more challenging exercises found in Chapter 8 such as mini squats and the clam.

Chapter 21: How To Progress Exercises

There are a few different ways you can progress exercises:

1) Repetitions: The simplest way to progress an exercise is to increase the number of repetitions that you do. As a general rule, once you can do 30 reps of an exercise easily, you are ready to move on to something more challenging

2) Weights: Another simple way to progress strengthening exercises is to add a weight (e.g. ankle weights, or simply wear a shoe). When you first do this, it is a good idea to reduce the number of repetitions you do of the exercise and gradually build them up again as the muscles are working harder. Don't be tempted to rush into using weights too quickly after a knee replacement.

3) Extras: Sometimes there are clever ways to increase the difficulty of an exercise e.g. adopting a different position. You will find advice on these with each exercise, if it is appropriate.

Getting The Best Results

I can't stress enough how important it is to start doing exercises before your knee replacement so you are in the best shape possible, and the importance of sticking with your rehab programme on a daily basis over the first few weeks and months after your operation. It really does make all the difference. In most cases, it is the people who follow their exercise programme religiously that get the best results. Here are my top tips:

1) Start Slow

Don't overdo things especially early on as it will do more harm than good. If an exercise is too difficult at the beginning, revisit it every week or so to find out when you are ready to add it in to your rehab programme.

2) Progress Slowly but Steadily

Aim to progress your exercises every 3-4 days e.g. increasing the number of repetitions, add weights or progress on to a more challenging exercise. As muscles strengthen and stretch, they need to be worked harder to improve further. Remember, each exercise is different so you will progress at different rates for different exercises – don't expect to be able to do the same number of reps for each exercise.

3) Be Consistent

Get into a regular habit of doing your knee exercises. Pick a regular time of the day, set an alarm, or link doing your exercises with a specific daily activity e.g. each time you have a cup of tea or eat a meal, do your exercises. This can make it much easier to remember.

4) Take a Break

Sometimes, doing exercises can get boring. Those first few weeks you really should be doing your exercises every day but after that, if you strength and movement is progressing well, have one day of the week where you take things easier to give yourself a break.

5) Variety is the Spice of Life

People often find it helps to split their exercises into two groups and do one lot at a time for a bit of variety. There is also usually more than one way to perform an exercise e.g. starting in a different position which can help keep things fresh. Or try exercising with someone else - that can be a great way to keep motivated.

6) Be Realistic

It takes time to build up strength and mobility. Whilst you should start to notice a difference after a few days, you are going to need to do exercises for a few months to really get the most benefit.

7) Acknowledge Progress

Every few weeks think back to where you were at the beginning of everything and see how far you've come – e.g. more movement, stronger, more flexible, able to do activities you couldn't do before, less pain etc. It really boosts your confidence. It can be hard to recognise progress from day to day, so stepping back can really help. Or ask those around you what they have noticed about your progress. It can really help to motivate you to keep going.

8) Think of the Goal

Remind yourself why you are doing each exercise – you are much more likely to stick with an exercise if you know how it is going to help you. Each of the knee exercises has an explanation of what it is aiming to achieve. And think what activities you are aiming to get back to, giving yourself a realistic plan of when you hope to restart.

9) Do it Right

Follow the exercise descriptions and every few days re-read them – I've had clients who have started off doing things slightly wrong and never noticed, so they haven't achieved the best results possible.

10) Sometimes Less is More

It is better to do less repetitions and perform knee exercises properly than it is to try and increase the number of repetitions so quickly that you lose the precision. And take things slowly. It is usually harder work for muscles to do exercises slowly, especially the hold part of the movement, than to rush through them quickly.

Chapter 22: Problems Following Surgery

Knee replacement problems are usually fairly minor and short lived, with approximately 90% of knee replacements being extremely successful[1]. But occasionally, problems do develop. All surgery carries risks and in the early days following surgery, things can feel uncomfortable.

General Risks Of Surgery

With any surgery, there are risks. These include bleeding and infection. Risks associated with anaesthesia include breathing problems and reactions to the medications. You doctor should discuss all of these with you at your pre-op appointment.

Specific risks for a knee replacement (partial or total) include:

1) Blood Clots: these can travel around the body and cause problems such as a heart attack or stroke. This is why you are given compression stockings to wear initially after your operation. You may also be given blood thinning medication depending on your history. Getting moving quickly after your operation helps reduce the risk of blood clots

2) Infection: usually at the operation site but the infection can spread around your body. In some cases, you may be given antibiotics after surgery to reduce this risk

3) Blood Vessel/Nerve Damage: may affect the sensation around the knee joint due to the incision

4) Pain Kneeling: you may need to kneel on a cushion

5) Complex Regional Pain Syndrome: rare problem with circulation and sensation leading to ongoing pain and swelling

Short Term Problems

Short term problems tend to be fairly minor and settle down within a few weeks. The most common short term problems are:

1) Pain

Once the anaesthesia wears off, the knee may feel sore as a result of the surgery both inside the knee and around the scar. It is really important to be taking effective pain relief to keep this under control. As I've already said, don't try and manage without medication too quickly. It is much better to take prescribed medication to keep the pain under control so you can start you rehab exercises and get up and about.

People usually find that very quickly the knee feels much better and actually less painful than before the operation as you no longer have the arthritis pain and the knee is able to move more freely. As you regain more movement and strength in the knee, the pain should decrease.

2) Numbness

Another common knee replacement problem people sometimes find is that it may also feel a bit numb around their scar – this can happen because some of the small nerves that supply feeling to the skin are cut during the operation. Nerves can take up to two years to fully heal so you may notice improvement up until then. Any continuing numbness after that time is unlikely to change.

3) Swelling

Swelling is one of the most common knee replacement problems. There is usually swelling around the knee for the first few days after surgery. The knee is initially bandaged to help reduce this. Once the bandage is removed, Tubigrip compression bandages can be used to help reduce the swelling and support the knee.

Keeping the leg elevated when you are lying down or sitting helps the excess fluid to drain away from the knee and reduce swelling.

Another thing that can help is using ice therapy. When used properly, this helps to slow the blood flow and any bleeding in the joint, reducing swelling. There are a number of different ways to apply ice. Cryocuffs are often used in hospitals and once you get home you can use an ice pack, making sure you are using it safely as we discussed earlier.

Movement and exercise is another great way to reduce swelling as it pumps the fluid out of the joint. However, you have to get the right balance. If you try and do too much too soon, you can actually make the swelling worse. Follow the guidance of your physical therapist.

4) Strange Noises

Sometimes people find that their knee makes funny creaking/cracking/popping noises after a knee replacement. This is usually nothing to worry about and tends to settle down within a few months as everything heals.

Longer Term Problems

Longer term knee replacement problems are rare but include:

1) Wear & Tear of the New Joint

The joint implants can gradually wear over time. 92% of partial knee replacements last at least twenty years and 85% of total knee replacements still work after 20 years[26]. As surgical techniques and implant designs develop, these figures should further improve

2) Loosening of the New Joint

The implant may become loose which can cause pain and limit mobility. If this happens with a partial knee replacement, you will probably require a total knee replacement. If this happens with a total knee replacement, you might need to have the surgery repeated, known as a revision knee replacement

3) Infection in the Knee Joint

This can occur years after surgery. The knee may become hot, red and swollen.

4) Persistent Stiffness

In some cases the knee can feel quite stiff and difficult to move after surgery due to the formation of adhesions inside the knee. During surgery, essential lubricating fluids in the knee sometimes evaporate. Whilst this isn't usually a problem, if they aren't replenished quickly then adhesions can develop which can be painful and severely limit movement. In most cases these adhesions will resolve with exercises and physical therapy. However, in some instances people require a MUA – manipulation-under-anaesthetic. This is a non-surgical procedure where you are put to sleep and the surgeon applies steady pressure to bend the knee and break through the adhesions. You are usually discharged the same day or the following day. Again, it is vital to start work on your rehab programme immediately to gain the maximum benefit from the procedure. A CPM (continuous passive motion) machine may be recommended by your surgeon. This is a machine that bends your knee up and down continuously for you. You can change the settings to increase the amount of flexion as the knee loosens. It is an adjunct to treatment, not a replacement for exercises – it is just as important to keep doing your exercises if you are using a CPM. Only around 4.5% of patients who have undergone a total knee replacement will require a MUA[27].

You will know if something is seriously wrong as the knee will become very painful, it may swell, and you may notice redness around the knee joint all of which may be accompanied by a fever. If this happens you should talk to your doctor immediately.

Chapter 23: Stats on Knee Replacements

Here are some interesting stats on knee replacements in the US[1]:

Knee replacements were the 14th most common in-patient procedure in 2009

The number of knee replacements increased by 84% between 1997 & 2007 per 10,000 population

5% of people have both knees replaced at the same time

Knee replacements are more common in women than men. The male:female percentage ratio for knee replacements in 2010 was 37:63

90% of patients experience dramatic reduction in their pain following a knee replacement

95% of patients report they are satisfied with their procedure

6% of patients required a revision knee replacement after 5 years, 12% after 10 years

Chapter 24: Closing Summary

I hope that you are now feeling empowered to manage your knee and that this book has answered your questions on arthritis and knee replacements. My hope is that with the information presented here, you will be able to better understand what is going on in your knee and how to take back control and get back to the life you want without pain stopping you.

If you would like any further information, please visit my website www.knee-pain-explained.com where there is a wealth of information of all aspects of knee pain including dedicated sections on both arthritis and knee replacements as well as knee pain diagnosis, common knee conditions and injuries, treatment options and anatomy.

I would love to hear how you have found this book – please do drop me a line via the contact form on the website www.knee-pain-explained.com.

If you enjoyed reading this book, I'd really appreciate it if you would take a couple of minutes to post a short review at Amazon. Intelligent reviews help other customers make better buying choices. And because I read all my reviews personally, they will help me to write better books in the future. Thanks for your support!

References

1) http://www.healthline.com/health/total-knee-replacement-surgery/statistics-infographic

2) http://www.ncbi.nlm.nih.gov/pmc/articles/PMC3766936/

3) http://www.ncbi.nlm.nih.gov/pmc/articles/PMC1753462/

4) http://www.ncbi.nlm.nih.gov/pmc/articles/PMC3291123/

5) http://www.cdc.gov/arthritis/basics/osteoarthritis.html

6) https://www.bjj.boneandjoint.org.uk/content/88-B/12/1549/T1.expansion.html

7) http://www.ncbi.nlm.nih.gov/pubmed/19333985

8) http://www.ncbi.nlm.nih.gov/pmc/articles/PMC2694558/

9) http://www.oarsijournal.com/article/S1063-4584%2813%2900763-2/abstract

10) http://www.wjgnet.com/2218-5836/pdf/v2/i5/37.pdf

11) http://onlinelibrary.wiley.com/doi/10.1002/art.21139/pdf

12) http://www.ncbi.nlm.nih.gov/pmc/articles/PMC2810544/

13) http://www.arthritis.org/living-with-arthritis/treatments/natural/supplements-herbs/guide/fish-oil.php

14) http://www.arthritis.org/living-with-arthritis/treatments/natural/supplements-herbs/guide/glucosamine.php

15) http://www.arthritis.org/living-with-arthritis/treatments/natural/supplements-herbs/osteoarthritis-hand-chondroitin-sulfate.php

16) http://www.arthritis.org/living-with-arthritis/treatments/natural/supplements-herbs/guide/sam-e.php

17) http://www.arthritis.org/living-with-arthritis/treatments/natural/supplements-herbs/guide/avocado-soybean.php

18) http://www.arthritis.org/living-with-arthritis/treatments/natural/supplements-herbs/guide/indian-frankincense.php

19) http://www.herbwisdom.com/herb-feverfew.html

20) http://www.arthritis.org/living-with-arthritis/treatments/natural/supplements-herbs/guide/ginger.php

21) http://www.besthealthmag.ca/best-you/home-remedies/natural-home-remedies-arthritis

22) http://www.disabled-world.com/medical/alternative/homeremedies/treating-arthritis-remedy.php

23)http://www.milk.co.uk/page.aspx?intpageid=327

24) http://www.anationinmotion.org/value/knee/

25)http://www.ncbi.nlm.nih.gov/pmc/articles/PMC2263116/

26) http://www.healthline.com/health/total-knee-replacement-surgery/outcomes-statistics-success-rate#1

27) http://www.em-consulte.com/en/article/288187

About The Author

Chloe Wilson worked as a physiotherapist in the UK for over 10 years. Training in Sheffield, UK, she went on to work in a number of different hospitals and health centres in Oxfordshire, England, as well as overseas in Uganda, East Africa.

She specialised in musculoskeletal physiotherapy including in-patient and out-patient trauma and orthopaedics. She ran the lower limb rehab team at the Horton Hospital, Oxfordshire and also worked in a GP commissioned triage service.

Her passion is to empower people and thoroughly involve them in the rehab process, which led her to creating the website, www.knee-pain-explained.com back in 2010. It was such a success that in 2013, she went on to develop a sister site, www.foot-pain-explored.com, with more in the pipeline for the near future.

It was following repeated requests from site visitors that she began to write books offering a greater depth and range of information to compliment the sites, for those who are looking for that bit more.

Chloe carried out a number of post graduate courses including the Society of Orthopaedic Medicine Lower Limb Course, Acupuncture, Trigger Points, Cognitive Behavioural Therapy and Pilates.

Chloe is director of Wilson Health Ltd, a UK company based in Oxfordshire, company number 9359622. Registered address 5 Minton Place, Victoria Road, Bicester, Oxon, OX26 6QB.

Printed in Great Britain
by Amazon